T0263411

Remote Monitoring and Physiologic Sensing Technologies

Editors

SAMUEL J. ASIRVATHAM
K.L. VENKATACHALAM
SURAJ KAPA

CARDIAC ELECTROPHYSIOLOGY CLINICS

www.cardiacEP.theclinics.com

Consulting Editors
RANJAN K. THAKUR
ANDREA NATALE

September 2013 • Volume 5 • Number 3

ELSEVIER

1600 John F. Kennedy Boulevard • Suite 1800 • Philadelphia, Pennsylvania, 19103-2899

http://www.theclinics.com

CARDIAC ELECTROPHYSIOLOGY CLINICS Volume 5, Number 3
September 2013 ISSN 1877-9182, ISBN-13: 978-0-323-18846-3

Editor: Barbara Cohen-Kligerman
Developmental Editor: Susan Showalter

Cardiac Electrophysiology Clinics (ISSN 1877-9182) is published quarterly by Elsevier Inc., 360 Park Avenue South, New York, NY 10010-1710. Months of issue are March, June, September, and December. Subscription prices are $191.00 per year for US individuals, $277.00 per year for US institutions, $100.00 per year for US students and residents, $214.00 per year for Canadian individuals, $309.00 per year for Canadian institutions, $273.00 per year for international individuals, $331.00 per year for international institutions and $143.00 per year for Canadian and foreign students/residents. To receive student/resident rate, orders must be accompanied by name of affiliated institution, date of term, and the signature of program/residency coordinator on institution letterhead. Orders will be billed at individual rate until proof of status is received. Foreign air speed delivery is included in all Clinics subscription prices. All prices are subject to change without notice. **POSTMASTER:** Send address changes to Cardiac Electrophysiology Clinics, Elsevier Health Sciences Division, Subscription Customer Service, 3251 Riverport Lane, Maryland Heights, MO 63043. **Customer Service: 1-800-654-2452 (US and Canada). From outside of the US and Canada, call 314-477-8871. Fax: 314-447-8029. E-mail: JournalsCustomerService-usa@elsevier.com (for print support); JournalsOnlineSupport-usa@elsevier.com (for online support).**

Reprints. For copies of 100 or more of articles in this publication, please contact the Commercial Reprints Department, Elsevier Inc., 360 Park Avenue South, New York, NY 10010-1710. Tel.: 212-633-3812; Fax: 212-462-1935; E-mail: reprints@elsevier.com.

Printed and bound by CPI Group (UK) Ltd, Croydon, CR0 4YY

Transferred to digital print 2012

Contributors

CONSULTING EDITORS

RANJAN K. THAKUR, MD, MPH, MBA, FHRS
Professor of Medicine and Director, Arrhythmia
Service, Thoracic and Cardiovascular Institute,
Sparrow Health System, Michigan State
University, Lansing, Michigan

ANDREA NATALE, MD, FACC, FHRS
Executive Medical Director, Texas Cardiac
Arrhythmia Institute, St David's Medical
Center, Austin, Texas; Consulting Professor,
Division of Cardiology, Stanford University,
Palo Alto, California; Adjunct Professor of
Medicine, Heart and Vascular Center, Case
Western Reserve University, Cleveland, Ohio;
Director, Interventional Electrophysiology,
Scripps Clinic, San Diego, California; Senior
Clinical Director, EP Services, California Pacific
Medical Center, San Francisco, California

EDITORS

SAMUEL J. ASIRVATHAM, MD
Professor of Medicine and Pediatrics,
Department of Internal Medicine and Pediatric
Cardiology, St Mary's Hospital, Mayo Clinic
College of Medicine, Rochester, Minnesota

SURAJ KAPA, MD
Senior Associate Consultant, Division of
Cardiology, Mayo Clinic College of Medicine,
Rochester, Minnesota

K.L. VENKATACHALAM, MD
Assistant Professor of Medicine, Department
of Internal Medicine, Division of Cardiology,
Mayo Clinic College of Medicine, Jacksonville,
Florida

AUTHORS

RIZWAN ALIMOHAMMAD, MD
Fellow, Division of Cardiology, Department of
Internal Medicine, Virginia Commonwealth
University School of Medicine and VCUHS
Medical Center, Richmond, Virginia

SAMUEL J. ASIRVATHAM, MD
Professor of Medicine and Pediatrics,
Department of Internal Medicine and
Pediatric Cardiology, St Mary's Hospital, Mayo
Clinic College of Medicine, Rochester,
Minnesota

DAVID G. BENDITT, MD
Professor of Medicine, Cardiovascular
Division, Cardiac Arrhythmia Center, University
of Minnesota School of Medicine, Minneapolis,
Minnesota

SARAH BONNELL, BS
Arrhythmia Institute, Valley Health System,
Columbia University College of Physicians and
Surgeons, New York, New York; Arrhythmia
Institute, Valley Health System, Columbia
University College of Physicians and Surgeons,
Ridgewood, New Jersey

HARAN BURRI, MD
University Hospital of Geneva, Geneva,
Switzerland

CASEY CABLE, MD
Department of Medicine, Mayo Clinic,
Jacksonville, Florida

YONG-MEI CHA, MD
Co-Director, Cardiac Implantable Device Lab,
Mayo Clinic, Rochester, Minnesota

ZHONGWEI CHENG, MD
Department of Cardiology, Peking Union
Medical College Hospital, Peking Union Medical
College and Chinese Academy of Medical
Sciences, Dongcheng District, Beijing, China

SANJAY DIXIT, MD
Associate Professor of Medicine, Section of
Cardiac Electrophysiology, Department of
Medicine, Hospital of the University of
Pennsylvania, Philadelphia, Pennsylvania

KENNETH A. ELLENBOGEN, MD
Kontos Professor of Medicine and Chair,
Division of Cardiology, Department of Internal
Medicine, Virginia Commonwealth University
School of Medicine and VCUHS Medical
Center, Richmond, Virginia

PAUL A. FRIEDMAN, MD
Director, Cardiac Implantable Device Lab,
Mayo Clinic, Rochester, Minnesota

JOSEPH J. GARD, MD
Fellow, Cardiovascular Medicine, Mayo Clinic,
Rochester, Minnesota

GAUTHAM KALAHASTY, MD
Associate Professor of Medicine, Division of
Cardiology, Department of Internal Medicine,
Virginia Commonwealth University School of
Medicine and VCUHS Medical Center,
Richmond, Virginia

SURAJ KAPA, MD
Senior Associate Consultant, Division of
Cardiology, Mayo Clinic College of Medicine,
Rochester, Minnesota

FRED M. KUSUMOTO, MD
Professor of Medicine, Mayo Clinic School of
Medicine; Director, Electrophysiology and
Pacing Services, Division of Cardiovascular
Disease, Department of Medicine, Mayo Clinic,
Jacksonville, Florida

RAHUL MAHAJAN
Virginia Commonwealth University School of
Medicine, Richmond, Virginia

JONATHAN P. MAN, MD
Section of Cardiac Electrophysiology,
Department of Medicine, University of
Pennsylvania, Philadelphia, Pennsylvania

SUNEET MITTAL, MD, FACC, FHRS
Associate Professor of Clinical Medicine,
Arrhythmia Institute, Valley Health System,
Columbia University College of Physicians and
Surgeons, New York, New York; Arrhythmia
Institute, Valley Health System, Columbia
University College of Physicians and Surgeons;
Director, Electrophysiology Laboratory,
The Valley Hospital, Ridgewood, New Jersey

SEJAL MORJARIA, MD
VCUHS Medical Center, Richmond, Virginia

ALEJANDRO A. RABINSTEIN, MD
Department of Neurology, Mayo Clinic,
Rochester, Minnesota

RAYMOND C.S. SEET, MD
Department of Medicine, Yong Loo Lin School
of Medicine, National University of Singapore,
Singapore

GREGORY E. SUPPLE, MD
Assistant Professor of Clinical Medicine,
Division of Cardiac Electrophysiology,
Department of Medicine, University of
Pennsylvania, Philadelphia, Pennsylvania

NIRAJ VARMA, MA, DM, FRCP
Cardiac Pacing and Electrophysiology,
Department of Cardiovascular Medicine,
Cleveland Clinic, Cleveland, Ohio

K.L. VENKATACHALAM, MD
Assistant Professor of Medicine, Department
of Internal Medicine, Division of Cardiology,
Mayo Clinic College of Medicine, Jacksonville,
Florida

PAUL J. WANG, MD, FACC, FHRS, FAHA
Professor, Cardiovascular Medicine, Stanford
University, Stanford, California

WILL W. XIONG, MD, PhD
Fellow in Clinical Cardiac Electrophysiology,
Cardiovascular Division, Cardiac Arrhythmia
Center, University of Minnesota School of
Medicine, Minneapolis, Minnesota

Contents

> Remote monitoring is an evolving technology that has already transformed the concept of cardiac rhythm monitoring. Clinical studies are now underway to determine the validity of remote monitoring with respect to patient outcome efficacy and societal efficacy. Beginning with the advent of the Holter monitor and progressing to today's fully automated remote interrogation systems, remote monitoring offers the clinician an unprecedented amount of data and responsibility.

> A variety of cardiac implantable electronic devices are used routinely in clinical practice, including implantable loop recorders, permanent pacemakers, implantable cardioverter-defibrillators (ICDs), cardiac resynchronization therapy-permanent pacemakers, and cardiac resynchronization therapy-ICDs. Following implantation, these devices require either in-office or remote follow-up. This article reviews the current guidelines for remote monitoring and follow-up of cardiac implantable electronic devices.

> Implanted devices such as pacemakers and cardiac defibrillators have become an established treatment for patients with symptomatic bradycardia or for those who are at risk for sudden cardiac death. Identification of arrhythmias is one of the most important functions of remote monitoring. Arrhythmias identified by a device may have important prognostic information. In addition to providing information on risk of thromboembolic events, remote monitoring of arrhythmias may have a use for evaluating efficacy of pharmacologic or nonpharmacologic therapy. Early identification of device problems, such as lead failures or accelerated battery depletion, is essential for maximizing the benefits of device therapy.

> This article reviews the most commonly used rate-adaptive sensor systems. Activity sensing (mainly accelerometer-based), minute ventilation, and closed-loop stimulation sensors using electrical bioimpedance are currently the primary systems.

Sensor blending and sensor cross-checking are the most important modalities of sensor combination for heart-rate adaptation. Also, sensors for monitoring heart failure have been developed with the objective of identifying heart-failure exacerbations earlier. Intrathoracic impedance, intracardiac ventricular impedance, and peak endocardial acceleration have been used for hemodynamic monitoring. Future hemodynamic sensors will reliably assess crucial hemodynamic variables such as preload, afterload, left ventricular ejection fraction, and stroke volume.

Sensors that reflect physical activity, heart rate variability, thoracic impedance, and myocardial ischemia monitoring may add importantly to the capabilities of implantable cardioverter defibrillators in patient management. Intracardiac monitoring of right ventricular systolic pulmonary artery pressure and left atrial pressure exhibits considerable promise in guiding therapy in the future. Monitoring these sensors might allow appropriate interventions to prevent heart failure and heart failure hospitalization and to detect early myocardial ischemia.

Intravascular leads are the most vulnerable component of conventional pacemakers and defibrillators. This article discusses the current state of technology for leadless cardiac devices in the treatment of bradycardia and for reducing sudden cardiac death caused by tachyarrhythmias.

Cardiac implantable electronic devices are increasing in prevalence. Conventionally, patients are monitored on a calendar-based in-person follow up schedule, and interim patient complaints prompt unanticipated hospital visits. In contrast, implantable devices with automatic remote monitoring capability provide a means for performing constant surveillance, with the ability to identify salient problems rapidly. This technology permits early detection of patient and/or system problems and resolution of cardiac complaints as and when they occur, without compulsory hospital visits.

Stroke patients undergo prolonged cardiac monitoring based on concern that those currently classified as having a cryptogenic cause and treated with antiplatelet therapy may actually have paroxysmal atrial fibrillation and merit anticoagulation for secondary stroke prevention. Technological advances have produced monitoring devices that can be applied to any patient, are capable of capturing electrocardiogram information accurately and continuously, and can relay critical data to the physician promptly. Even if monitors can detect arrhythmias with perfect accuracy, it has not been demonstrated in clinical trials that more strokes can be prevented by anticoagulation guided by the findings of prolonged rhythm monitoring.

Atrial fibrillation has been shown to increase the risk of thromboembolic complications, heart failure, and death. Establishing a diagnosis of atrial fibrillation in these patients may result in changes of management. The utility of different types of remote monitoring in diagnosing atrial fibrillation depends on the length and type of remote monitor used, with monitored telemetry giving the highest yield and short-term Holter monitoring the lowest. The choice of monitoring needs to take into account the data sought, the arrhythmia burden, and the cost.

Patients with cardiac conditions represent the largest group monitored using wireless technology. Over the past 50 years, the technology has evolved to encompass the measurement and tracking of multiple physiologic parameters, allowing clinicians to monitor the cardiac status of patients automatically and through patient-initiated downloads. This article reviews the technologic advances that have been made in this field and covers pivotal study results that demonstrate the usefulness of this approach in the diagnosis and treatment of cardiac arrhythmias and heart failure. Potential exciting new applications of this technology also are discussed.

Cardiac monitors collect and transmit information about heart rate and rhythm. Physiologic sensors in implantable devices allow clinicians to remotely monitor heart failure status. Wireless networks will evolve to transmit data more effectively. Improved algorithms may improve arrhythmia recognition by diagnostic monitors. Applications for smartphones can offer novel and cost-effective means to medically monitor patients. The evolution of physiologic sensors may advance cardiac monitoring beyond heart rate and rhythm alone. Sensors may assist in several areas. The usefulness of these innovations will require validation clinically as well as consideration of cost and who will manage the data.

Remote monitoring of cardiac parameters will continue to play an important clinical role in the diagnosis and treatment of cardiovascular disease. The volume of clinical data produced by the increasing use of this technology will need to be managed using efficient approaches to the processing of such data. The technologies will need to be thoroughly and continually tested in a clinical setting to confirm their relevance and to prevent clinicians from being misled by the physiologic data.

CARDIAC ELECTROPHYSIOLOGY CLINICS

Foreword
Health Care Challenge—Do It Better, Cheaper, and Faster

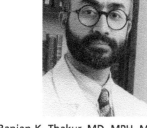
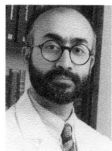

Ranjan K. Thakur, MD, MPH, MBA, FHRS   Andrea Natale, MD, FACC, FHRS
Consulting Editors

As health care has become the largest sector of the economy in most developed countries (18% of the US gross domestic product), it is under increasing pressure to become more efficient (better and cheaper). While we have many social and political issues related to healthcare, technological advancements will enable more efficient delivery in many instances. With improvements in drugs, devices, procedures, information technologies, and so on, not only will we be able to deliver health care better and cheaper but also we may be able to do it faster.

Implantable heart rhythm devices have undergone a revolution in our lifetime. Not only are these devices getting smaller and smarter (pacemakers and defibrillators [ICDs]), but technological advances have also opened up entirely new avenues. The implantable loop recorder, initially used for the diagnosis of unexplained syncope, will likely revolutionize monitoring for cardiac arrhythmias, as, for example, in patients with cryptogenic strokes or after catheter ablation for atrial fibrillation (AF).

Traditionally, patients with permanent pacemakers and defibrillators have been followed periodically in clinics. Not only is this expensive, but no information is available between visits. A patient with a pacemaker may go into AF the day after a clinic visit and subsequently sustain a stroke, yet the physician may be in the dark and unable to do anything because of a lack of information. Techno-

logical advances have allowed remote monitoring of pacemakers and defibrillators, which allows interventions to avert problems. For example, it is now possible to know that a pacemaker or ICD patient has developed AF almost immediately and to institute anticoagulation when appropriate to avert a stroke. Similarly, it is possible to learn quickly that an ICD patient has been shocked multiple times as well as the cause of those shocks, and take appropriate steps to prevent further problems.

These technological advances also raise new questions, such as who will pay for them and medical-legal issues. In due course, these questions will be resolved.

This issue of *Cardiac Electrophysiology Clinics*, edited by Drs Asirvatham, Venkatachalam, and Kapa, focuses on Remote Monitoring and Physiologic Sensing Technologies. They have addressed the aforementioned issues and also provided a historical perspective on remote cardiac monitoring, sensor technologies for pacemakers and ICDs, leadless pacing, and defibrillator technologies.They also consider future trends in the evolution of remote monitoring and physiologic sensing technologies. We congratulate them for tackling a rapidly evolving field and summarizing the current state of knowledge regarding today's relevant issues.

Technological advancements have always led to human progress—longer, healthier, and more

Card Electrophysiol Clin 5 (2013) ix–x
http://dx.doi.org/10.1016/j.ccep.2013.07.002
1877-9182/13/$ – see front matter © 2013 Published by Elsevier Inc.

productive lives. We should understand, embrace, and improve the new tools, so that we can deliver health care "better, cheaper, and faster."

Ranjan K. Thakur, MD, MPH, MBA, FHRS
Sparrow Thoracic and Cardiovascular Institute
Michigan State University
1200 East Michigan Avenue, Suite 580
Lansing, MI 48912, USA

Andrea Natale, MD, FACC, FHRS
Texas Cardiac Arrhythmia Institute
Center for Atrial Fibrillation at
St. David's Medical Center
1015 East 32nd Street, Suite 516
Austin, TX 78705, USA

E-mail addresses:
thakur@msu.edu (R.K. Thakur)
andrea.natale@stdavids.com (A. Natale)

Preface

Remote Monitoring and Physiologic Sensing Technologies

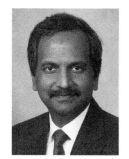 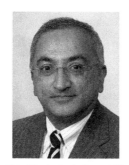 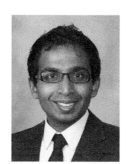

Samuel J. Asirvatham, MD   K.L. Venkatachalam, MD   Suraj Kapa, MD

Editors

Modern methods of cardiovascular monitoring encompass a vast array of sensing, transmitting, and processing technologies that have variable utility depending on the physiologic parameter and disease process being evaluated. As the population continues to age and technology improves—both by miniaturization of existing hardware and by improvement in the ability to collect, process, and transmit real-time information for a variety of physiologic variables—the options to treat patients in the ambulatory setting will continue to evolve. The cardiac electrophysiologist will often be responsible for the choice of monitoring technology, the implantation or implementation of it, and the interpretation of the resultant data. Furthermore, with improved availability of these technologies, both physicians and patients will continue to encounter an increasing ability and desire to treat or monitor patients at home, which will require a thorough understanding of current options and their corresponding indications

and limitations. Thus, a thorough understanding of remote monitoring technologies and the data underlying their use is critical to the modern electrophysiologist.

In this issue of *Cardiac Electrophysiology Clinics*, we focus on remote monitoring, including the history underlying its development, the current state of the technology, and potential future routes of development and study. Also found in this issue are current data on the utility of existing remote monitoring technologies in disease processes ranging from atrial fibrillation to stroke. Also presented are state-of-the-art, not yet clinically available technologies to widen the scope of the reader on what the future of these technologies may hold. Thus, through this edition of the *Cardiac Electrophysiology Clinics*, the reader may expect to attain a comprehensive outlook on the current state of remote monitoring and physiologic sensing technologies along with perspectives on how they

Card Electrophysiol Clin 5 (2013) xi–xii
http://dx.doi.org/10.1016/j.ccep.2013.07.001
1877-9182/13/$ – see front matter © 2013 Published by Elsevier Inc.

may be utilized in current and future clinical practice and research.

Samuel J. Asirvatham, MD
Department of Internal Medicine and
Pediatric Cardiology
St Mary's Hospital
Mayo Clinic College of Medicine
200 First Street SW
Rochester, MN 55905, USA

K.L. Venkatachalam, MD
Department of Internal Medicine
Division of Cardiology
Mayo Clinic College of Medicine
4500 San Pablo Road, Davis 7
Jacksonville, FL 32224, USA

Suraj Kapa, MD
Division of Cardiology
Mayo Clinic College of Medicine
200 First Street SW
Rochester, MN 55905, USA

E-mail addresses:
asirvatham.samuel@mayo.edu (S.J. Asirvatham)
venkat.Kl@mayo.edu (K.L. Venkatachalam)
Kapa.Suraj@mayo.edu (S. Kapa)

A Brief History of Remote Cardiac Monitoring

Gautham Kalahasty, MD[a],*, Rizwan Alimohammad, MD[a],
Rahul Mahajan[b], Sejal Morjaria, MD[c],
Kenneth A. Ellenbogen, MD[a]

KEYWORDS

- Cardiac rhythm • Remote monitoring • Holter monitor • Transtelephonic monitoring
- Intermittent recorders

KEY POINTS

- Remote monitoring (RM) is an evolving technology that has already transformed the concept of cardiac rhythm monitoring.
- Clinical studies are now underway to determine the validity of remote monitor with respect to patient outcome efficacy and societal efficacy.
- Beginning with the advent of the Holter monitor and progressing to today's fully automated remote interrogation systems, RM offers the clinician an unprecedented amount of data and responsibility.

Remote cardiac monitoring refers to cardiac monitoring that is not conducted in clinical settings such as a hospital, clinic, or doctor's office. Multiple aspects of cardiovascular (CV) physiology can be monitored, including ambulatory blood pressure, ischemia, QT interval, heart rate variability, weight, blood pressure, cardiac rhythm, and volume status, to name a few. This article focuses on the history of cardiac rhythm monitoring, with an emphasis on the remote monitoring (RM) of cardiac rhythm management devices (CRMDs), including permanent pacemakers, implantable cardioverter-defibrillators (ICDs), cardiac resynchronization therapy devices, and implantable loop records (ILRs). Although they were conceived during different decades, the technologies of Holter monitoring, transtelephonic monitoring (TTM), event monitors, and RM have all advanced in parallel with each other and along with advances in computer (storage and analysis) and communication technologies. In addition, current technology is blurring the lines between these previously distinct diagnostic technologies. Consider for example, the Holter monitor, capable of recording continuously for up to 72 hours. Mobile cardiac outpatient telemetry (MCOT, CardioNet Inc) is a type of event monitor that can provide similar recording for more than 1 week. New wireless technologies, such as wireless LAN and sensor networks, for telecardiology purposes give new possibilities for monitoring of vital parameters with wearable biomedical sensors as well as for CRMDs. Patients now have the freedom to be mobile and still be under continuous monitoring.[1]

EARLY HISTORY

External cardiac monitoring begins with the British physiologist, Dr Augustus Waller M.D. who published the first electrocardiogram (ECG) in 1887 (**Fig. 1**). Dr Waller's simple apparatus used a mercury capillary electrometer to measure fluctuations

Disclosures: The authors have nothing to disclose.
a Division of Cardiology, Department of Internal Medicine, Virginia Commonwealth University School of Medicine and VCUHS Medical Center, PO Box 980053, Richmond, VA 23298-0053, USA; b Virginia Commonwealth University School of Medicine, Richmond, VA 23298, USA; c VCUHS Medical Center, Richmond, VA 23298, USA
* Corresponding author.
E-mail address: gkalahasty@mcvh-vcu.edu

Card Electrophysiol Clin 5 (2013) 275–282
http://dx.doi.org/10.1016/j.ccep.2013.06.002

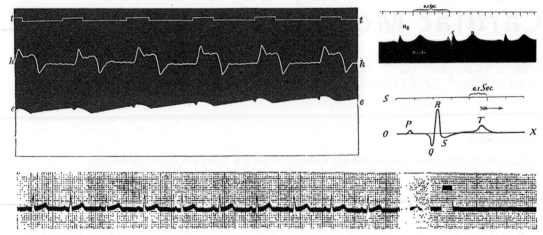

Fig. 1. Top left panel: first-published ECG using the capillary electrometer. The bottom waveform in white reflects measured deflections representing electrical activity. Top right panel: Einthoven's ECG recordings using capillary electrometer. Deflections of the electrometer waveform were referred to by letters A–E. Middle panel: correction of the capillary electrometer measurements using Einthoven's calculations allowed determination of a more accurate potential waveform. The corrected deflections came to be known by the letters P–T that persist to today. Bottom panel: ECG recordings using the refined string galvanometer, which allowed for potential measurements with a much faster frequency response and look much closer to modern ECGs. (*From* Waller AG. A demonstration on man of electromotive changes accompanying the heart's beat. J Physiol 1887;8:229–34; and Einthoven W. Die galvanometrische Registrierung des menschlichen Elektrokardiogramms, zugleich eine Beurteilung der Anwendung des Kapillar-Elektrometers in der Physiologie. Pflügers Arch 1903;99:472–80.)

in potential across a pair of leads, one strapped to the front of the chest and one strapped to the back.[2] Even with such an apparatus, his initial recordings showed deflections in surface potential and were able to demonstrate that electrical events preceded mechanical events by a measurable delay. Public demonstrations of Waller's work often involved his famous patient "Jimmy", his bulldog who would patiently stand with feet in jars of saline attached to electrodes. Among the observers of these demonstrations was the Danish physiologist Dr Willem Einthoven, considered by many to be the father of electrocardiography. Einthoven recognized many of the limitations of the capillary electrometer and developed several important advancements, including calculations to correct for waveform distortions caused by the electrometer and refinement of the string galvanometer (see **Fig. 1**),[3] originally invented by Ader.[4] These and other improvements by Einthoven led to the development of the first practical electrocardiograph (ECG) and his receiving of the Nobel Prize in Medicine in 1924 for the invention of the practical ECG.

MODERN HISTORY

Further maturation of technology allowed miniaturization of many of the components. Einthoven's original apparatus involved large instruments weighing several hundred pounds and necessitated multiple operators. In the succeeding years, the ECG was commercialized, miniaturized, and became a useful hospital tool in patient care.

By 1949, biophysicist Dr Norman "Jeff" Holter of Montana was attempting the first truly RM of cardiac surface potentials.[5] His initial device transmitted a 2-lead ECG by radio signals and was housed in a crude backpack weighing almost 85lbs (**Fig. 2**).[6] Within a few years, this device had been miniaturized down to a 2.6lb amplifier and transmitter.[7] Within 10 years, further miniaturization and refinements became possible with the start of the transistor age, and the device eventually abandoned radio transmission for local data storage on magnetic tape. By 1961, the Holter monitor was emerging a potential tool, and it quickly was adopted into clinical use where it became a lasting instrument for ambulatory monitoring. The first commercially available ambulatory ECG device was manufactured in 1962 (deliveries commencing in 1963) by Del Mar Engineering Laboratories under the name Avionics Research Products Corporation.[8] Once a recording was made, it could be played back and analyzed at 60X speed allowing a 24-hour recording to be analyzed in as little as 24 minutes. Magnetic tapes could record only 2 channels that were prone to recording limitations such as wow, flutter, tape head misalignment, as well as mechanical malfunctions. These

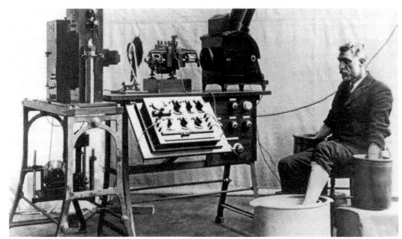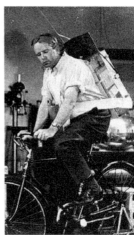

Fig. 2. Left: miniaturized commercial "table top" model of ECG apparatus using Einthoven's string galvanometer. Right: the first Holter monitor transmitted and ECG using radio signals. It weighed roughly 85 lbs and could be worn as a backpack. ([Left]: *From* Barron SL. Development of the electrocardiograph in Great Britain. Br Med J 1950;1:720; with permission. [Right]: Lot 18 Holter Research Foundation Photo Collection, Montana Historical Society Photograph Archives. *Courtesy of* Montana Historical Society, Helena, MT; with permission.)

issues were eliminated with the use of a PCMCIA type II digital recorder that acquired three leads of 8-bit data on a removable flash memory device. As the cost and size of greater memory capacity has decreased, digital recording has improved significantly in a few short years. Capable of recording as many as 12 leads, digital recorders can sample and store at very high rates with remarkable resolution for very long periods of time. Digital devices not only improve the capacity and accuracy of the recording but also allow for interface to more sophisticated software analysis. These software algorithms are used to reject artifact and screen for arrhythmias and other findings to flag for review by the technician and physician. More complex analyses such as heart rate variability can be performed as well. Although the Holter monitor remains an important clinical tool in today's practice, it is still limited in the overall duration of its recording. If the patient's symptoms are infrequent, a Holter monitor becomes an ineffective diagnostic tool. Another disadvantage of Holter monitors is the need to return the device for processing and analysis after each use. Even if a clinical event occurred during the study, the data needs to be screened, reviewed and correlated to the event. The data analysis is not done in real-time. Newer technologies include wearable patches that record the ECG for up to 7 days; they can be removed from the patient's body and mailed in for analysis.

TTM is a technology introduced in the early 1970s and has been, until this decade, the predominant method of remote pacemaker follow-up. It is also the basis for arrhythmia surveillance for the first generation of patient-activated event monitors.[9] This technology converts ECG information into sound, to communicate over telephone lines to a decoding machine, which changes the sound back into a "rhythm strip". TTM is discussed again later in this article.

Event monitors are another category of devices that are used to remotely assess cardiac rhythm abnormalities. **Box 1** summarizes the categories of available devices. Devices are categorized according to whether they monitor cardiac rhythm intermittently or continuously and whether they are worn externally or implanted. The technologies that have resulted in the advancement of these devices are the same as those that are responsible for the advancement of the Holter monitor. These include digital recording and storage, transtelephonic transmission, and software analysis of data.

Box 1
Categories of event monitors

Patient-activated or event-activated devices

- Presymptom memory loop recorders (attended and unattended)
- Implantable presymptom memory loop recorders
- Post-symptom recorders (attended or unattended)

Real-time continuous attended cardiac monitoring

The largest category in use today is the patient-activated/event-activated intermittent recorders (presymptom loop and post-symptoms recorders). Data from these devices are transmitted by phone to a doctor's office, clinic, hospital, or an independent diagnostic testing facility (IDTF). Service providers for these devices offer attended monitoring through their IDTFs. The standard external loop recorder (ELR) also uses memory loop recording capable of storing several minutes of data until it requires transmission to a monitoring center. The patient must signal an event to acquire data. Asymptomatic episodes (ie, some patients with atrial fibrillation) need an auto-trigger ELR. These also have a looping memory system. These recorders frequently auto-activate for false events or artifact, filling the memory and requiring the patient to perform frequent transmissions. Both these types of ELRs require the patient to perform a transtelephonic transmission to the monitoring center. Post-symptoms event recorders are hand-held devices that have no chest electrodes. These monitors do not have the memory loops of presymptoms recorders and can therefore record the rhythm that occurs only at trigger. The patient applies the monitor directly to the chest during the symptoms. Although they provide good correlation to patient symptoms and rhythm, they can miss clinical arrhythmias if the patient does not perform or cannot perform the needed steps. Most monitors are placed over the patient's chest, but several monitors exist that record the ECG from wrist bands similar in location to wearing a wristwatch.

Real-time *continuous* attended remote cardiac monitoring systems automatically record and transmit arrhythmic event data from ambulatory patients to personnel at a clinic, hospital, or, in most cases, an IDTF. The technicians at these IDTFs are trained to interpret cardiac arrhythmias and contact clinicians and/or patients based on preset parameters. The first generations of these monitors require the patient to take the device to a base station in the patient's home, which is linked to a land-based phone line. Newer devices have a built-in cellular telephone that automatically transmits events to the monitoring center virtually regardless of the patient location. The ability to respond immediately to clinical events as they occur is the major advantage of these systems.

ILRs perform the same function of external recorders but are implanted and are typically used for much longer periods of time. The Transoma Medical Sleuth was a programmable device with a wireless system that could transmit ECG data to an RM center. The Transoma Medical Co went out of business before this product reached significant clinical use. The currently available ILRs are manufactured by Medtronic Inc (Reveal) and St. Jude Medical Inc (Confirm). Neither of these devices has wireless technology and requires an in-office interrogation or a home RM unit (Medtronic Carelink or St. Jude Medical Merlin).

Initial implanted cardiac pacemakers required very close follow-up, including at least weekly 12 hour sessions for recharging of batteries via external induction. Improvements in battery technology allowed for long-term ambulatory devices. Almost immediately, methods for RM of cardiac events and device functions were explored. Initial efforts consisted of devices similar to Holter monitors that provided short-term recording of ambulatory ECGs. The recorded data were then reviewed in an office visit where it could be reviewed at 60x speeds. By the 1970s, TTM was providing an alternate means of monitoring.[10] Initially, the use of TTM was generally applied only for scheduled checks for monitoring the longevity of implanted pacemakers or for confirmation of symptomatic arrhythmias during checks initiated by the patient.[11] Although the clinical use of TTM further expanded to eventually include detection of more subtle pacemaker malfunction than battery depletion, including problems with sensing or capture, lead malfunctions, and even transtelephonic device programming,[12] TTM's adequacy as the sole form of follow-up for the first years following implantation of a pacemaker has been questioned.[13] TTM ICD interrogation was first reported in the early 1990s.[14] Transmitted data included programmed VT/VF detection criteria and therapies, battery status, charge time, episode counters, and therapy logs. In this study, there was complete accuracy of TTM data when compared to data obtained during standard in-office follow-up. Despite improvements in the technology including expansion of TTM use to ICDs (uncommon), the real-time nature of TTM interrogation limited it as a useful tool only for detection of pacemaker malfunction and significant arrhythmias.[15] Further studies have called into question its utility in detecting more than pulse generator failure, battery depletion, and lead failure[16] and have demonstrated its inferiority compared with in-office visits.[17] Thus, the data supporting the efficacy of TTM for pacemaker and ICD follow-up are mixed. The other inherent disadvantage of TTM is its reliance on the active cooperation of the patient who has to place a special device over his/her pacemaker or ICD.

In the 2008 PREFER clinical trial, the efficacy of the emerging technologies for RM compared favorably to TTM. This study concluded that remote pacemaker interrogation follow-up detects actionable events that are potentially important, more quickly and more frequently than TTM recordings. It also found the use of TTM for pacemaker follow-up to be of little value except for battery status determinations.[18]

MODERN REMOTE MONITORING

A combination of advancements within pacemakers and ICDs, cellular technology, and internet technologies have all driven and contributed to the development of the modern RM systems. Both pacemakers and ICDs are now able to store large amounts of arrhythmia data (ie, atrial fibrillation burden) and physiologic data (ie, transthoracic impedance: Optivol Medtronic, Inc) as well as basic information about lead integrity and device status. The usefulness of the information is dependent on its timely availability to clinicians.

Most of the CRMDs are also enabled with a radiofrequency transmitter that facilitates both in-office and RM. Medical Device Radiocommunications Service (MedRadio) dates back to 1999 when the FCC established the Medical Implant Communication Service (MICS). At that time, the FCC set aside 3 MHz of spectrum at 402 to 405 MHz for medical implant devices. This allowed for the development of the first RM system in 2001, Biotronik's Home Monitoring (HM). That same year, the first pacemaker capable of RM was implanted at Stanford University. By 2003, the first internet-based RM system was introduced along with compatible wireless and cellular transmitters. By 2006, the Centers for Medicare and Medicaid Service (CMS) approved a favorable reimbursement structure for RM and follow-up further incentivizing the acceptance of RM. In 2009, the FCC created the Medical Device Radiocommunications Service (MedRadio) in the 401 to 406 MHz range. The creation of the MedRadio Service incorporated the existing MICS spectrum at 402 to 405 MHz and added additional spectrum at 401 to 402 MHz and 405 to 406 MHz for a total of 5 MHz of spectrum for implanted devices as well as devices worn on the actual body.

Table 1 summarizes the currently available RM systems according to manufacturer. Each system is proprietary and works only with the associated devices. Biotronik's HM is the most extensively

Table 1
Remote monitoring systems from major manufacturers

	Biotronik	Medtronic	Boston Scientific	St. Jude Medical
Name	Home Monitoring	Carelink	Latitude	Merlin House Call Plus
FDA approval	2001	2005	2006	2007
Portable/ stationary	Portable	Stationary	Stationary	Stationary
Operation	Automatic	Patient-initiated and automatic	Patient-initiated and automatic	Automatic and patient-initiated
Devices monitored	ICD, PPM, CRT-P, CRT-D (all wireless)	ICD, CRT (PPMs and ILRs required wanded download)	ICD, CRT (no PPM) Wanded-operation and wireless	ICD, PPM, CRT-P and CRT-D (all wireless)
Technology	Cellular or landline	Landline	Landline	Landline or cellular
Event notification	Website; fax; e-mail; SMS	Website; phone; e-mail; SMS	Website; fax; phone	Website; fax; phone; SMS
Alert programming	Remote	Requires patient presence	Remote	Requires patient presence
Heart failure sensor	HRV	OptiVol	Weight, blood pressure	HRV

Abbreviations: CRT-D, cardiac resynchronization defibrillator; CRT-P, cardiac resynchronization therapy pacemaker; FDA, Food and Drug Administration; HRV, heart rate variability; ICD, implantable cardioverter-defibrillator; PPM, pacemaker; SMS, short message service.

Adapted from Ellenbogen K, Wilkoff B, Lau CP, editors. Clinical cardiac pacing, defibrillation, and resynchronization therapy. 4th edition. Philadelphia: Saunders; 2011; with permission.

studied system (see later discussion). There are significant differences between the systems with respect to patient involvement, alerts, transmission technology, and portability. Once data are transferred from the patient's device to the transmitter or base station, it is encrypted and uploaded via landline or cellular line to a secure central server maintained by the individual manufacturer. The standards for transmission are exceptionally high with no significant loss of data packets.[1]

One fundamental difference in the available systems is the degree of automation. This is a feature that truly distinguishes RM from scheduled TTMs. Automatic RM was pioneered by Biotronik (HM). The patient needs to be within 6 feet of the transceiver for it to link with the device and receive data on a scheduled basis. The data are then automatically transferred via cellular technology and sent to the physician on a prioritized basis. Customizable alerts can be programmed individually. Data acquisition and transmission are performed completely independent of the patient and physician. HM is also the most extensively studied system with clinical data supporting its reliability, accuracy, and early notification ability. It has also been shown to have a low energy cost with respect to battery depletion and is not susceptible to electromagnetic interference. The transceiver is a fully mobile unit and will work worldwide.

In contrast, Medtronic Inc, Boston Scientific Inc, and St Jude Medical Inc each have RM systems that require some degree of a patient-initiated follow-up. The patient must interact with the transceiver (apply the wand and/or initiate interrogation) and coordinate with clinic personnel on a scheduled basis.

As mentioned earlier, HM is an example of a clinically, well-studied RM system. In 2010, The Lumos-T Safely Reduces Routine Office Device Follow-Up (TRUST) trial tested the hypothesis that remote home monitoring with automatic daily surveillance (HM) is safe and effective for ICD follow-up and enables rapid physician evaluation of significant events.[19] In total, 1339 patients underwent 2:1 randomization to HM or conventional follow-up. Follow-up checks occurred at 3, 6, 9, 12, and 15 months after implantation. HM was used before office visits at 3 and 15 months in the HM group. At 6, 9, and 12 months, HM not only was used but also was followed by office visits if necessary. Conventional patients were evaluated with office visits only. Scheduled office visits and unscheduled evaluations, incidence of morbidity, and time elapsed from first event occurrence in each patient to physician evaluation were tracked for each group. The primary goal of the study was to assess the number of total in-hospital device

evaluations in HM compared with conventional care and to assess the safety of the remote follow-up method. RM reduced total hospital encounters for device interrogation by 45%. More than 90% of scheduled checks were nonactionable and did not necessitate an in-person device clinic encounter. The secondary endpoint compared detection times of clinically significant events, assessed by time from event onset (from device diagnostics) to physician evaluation of first occurrence of arrhythmia (AF, VT, VF, and SVT) in individual patients. Detection was advanced by more than 30 days compared to the conventional group. It is data from this trial that led the FDA to issue the unique and specific labeling to the Biotronik HM system as the only RM approved to replace in-office device follow-up.

Other clinical studies support the use of RM. In 2010, The CONNECT (Clinical Evaluation of Remote Notification to Reduce Time to Clinical Decision) trial looked at the value of wireless RM with automatic clinician alert.[20] The primary objective was to determine if wireless RM with automatic clinician alerts reduces the time from a clinical event to a clinical decision in response to arrhythmias, CV disease progression, or device-related issues compared to patients receiving standard in-office care. The secondary objective was to compare the rates of CV health care utilization between patients in the remote and in-office groups. Health care utilization data were defined as all CV-related hospitalizations, emergency department visits, and clinic or office visits. This study was a multicenter, prospective, randomized evaluation involving 1997 patients from 136 clinical sites who underwent insertion of an ICD (including cardiac resynchronization therapy devices) and were observed for 15 months. The overall findings of the study were similar to those of the TRUST trial. This study demonstrated that wireless RM allows clinicians to make clinical decisions 17.4 days sooner when compared with the in-office group. RM patients with atrial tachycardia/atrial fibrillation events had a reduced median time from arrhythmia onset to a responsive clinical action (3 days vs 24 days). The health care utilization data revealed a decrease in mean length of stay per cardiovascular hospitalization from 4 days (in-office group) to 3.3 days in the RM group ($P<.002$). The Medtronic Carelink system was used in this study and, unlike HM, is an entirely patient-initiated system. Once the system was activated, a successful transmission led to a clinician viewing the data within 1.5 days 70% of the time. This study highlights the need for the supporting infrastructure within individual clinical setting that is adequate to respond to the incoming data.

The impact of RM on mortality was studied in the ALTITUDE trial.[21] This project was an independent clinical study initiated in 2008 and prospectively analyzed data from Boston Scientific's LATITUDE RM system. The study asserted that there is a mortality benefit to patients followed on the RM system compared with those undergoing traditional in-office follow-up. Despite its novel conclusions, this study has major limitations preventing its generalization. Among these limitations are the absence of randomization and major lack of clinical profile data, specifically comorbid conditions.

There are many unresolved questions regarding RM including those related to quality assurance as well as medical-legal issues. Data currently reside on servers owned by the manufacturers. Data ownership and privacy issues are unresolved. Practical issues related to office staffing and the monitoring of incoming data need to be decided at the individual clinic level. The HRS expert consensus statement regarding the monitoring of CRMs address many of these issues, and the reader is referred to this document for complete details.[22]

SUMMARY

As with all technologies it is interesting to consider remote cardiac monitoring in the conceptual framework proposed by Fryback and Thornbury.[23] This 6-tiered hierarchical model suggests an approach to analyze the efficacy of a diagnostic technology. The 6 levels are

- Level 1: Technical efficacy
- Level 2: Diagnostic accuracy efficacy
- Level 3: Diagnostic thinking efficacy (percentage of patients for whom the test was helpful in making a diagnosis)
- Level 4: Therapeutic efficacy (percentage of patients for whom the test resulted in a change in management)
- Level 5: Patient outcome efficacy (percentage of patients improved with the test than without the test)
- Level 6: Societal efficacy (cost-effectiveness analysis from a societal viewpoint)

RM is an evolving technology that has already transformed the concept of cardiac rhythm monitoring. Despite the many unanswered question regarding RM, clinical data presented earlier establish its progression solidly through level 4 of the Fryback framework. Clinical studies are now underway to determine the validity of RM with respect to patient outcome efficacy (level 5) and societal efficacy (level 6).

RM of cardiac rhythm has advanced remarkably since the days of Waller and Einthoven. Beginning with the advent of the Holter monitor and progressing to today's fully automated remote interrogation systems, RM now offers the clinician an unprecedented amount of data and responsibility. The efficacious use of this data is a subject for another article in medical history.

REFERENCES

1. Kumar S, Kambhatla K, Hu F, et al. Ubiquitous computing for remote cardiac patient monitoring: a survey. Int J Telemed Appl 2008;19.
2. Waller AG. A demonstration on man of electromotive changes accompanying the heart's beat. J Physiol 1887;8:229–34.
3. Einthoven W. Die galvanometrische Registrierung des menschlichen Elektrokardiogramms, zugleich eine Beurteilung der Anwendung des Kapillar-Elektrometers in der Physiologie. Pflügers Arch 1903;99:472–80.
4. Ader C. Sur un nouvel appareil enregistreur pour cables sous-marins. Compt Rendus Acad Sci 1897; 124:1440–2.
5. Holter NJ, Generelli JA. Remote recording of physiologic data by radio. Rocky Mt Med J 1949;46: 747–51.
6. Corday E. Historical vignette celebrating the 30th anniversary of diagnostic ambulatory electrocardiographic monitoring and data reduction systems. J Am Coll Cardiol 1991;17(1):286–92.
7. Barold S. Norman J. "Jeff" Holter-"Father" of ambulatory ECG monitoring. J Interv Card Electrophysiol 2005;14(2):117–8.
8. Del Mar B. The history of clinical Holter monitoring. Ann Noninvasive Electrocardiol 2005;10(2):226–30.
9. Grodman RS, Capone RJ, Most AS. Arrhythmia surveillance by transtelephonic monitoring: comparison with Holter monitoring in symptomatic ambulatory patients. Am Heart J 1979;4:459–64.
10. Peter T, Luxton M, McDonald R, et al. Personal telephone electrocardiogram transmitter. Lancet 1973; 302:1110–2.
11. Hasin Y, David D, Rogel S. Diagnostic and therapeutic assessment by telephone electrocardiographic monitoring of ambulatory patients. Br Med J 1976; 2(6036):609–12.
12. Griffin JC, Schuenemeyer TD, Hess KR. Pacemaker follow-up: its role in the detection and correction of pacemaker malfunction. Pacing Clin Electrophysiol 1986;9:387–91.
13. Vallario LE, Leman RB, Gillette PC. Pacemaker follow-up and adequacy of Medicare guidelines. Am Heart J 1988;116:11–5.
14. Anderson MH, Paul VE, Jones S, et al. Transtelephonic interrogation of the implantable cardioverter

defibrillator. Pacing Clin Electrophysiol 1998;21: 1893–900.

15. Gessman LJ, Vielbig RE, Waspe LE, et al. Accuracy and clinical utility of transtelephonic pacemaker follow-up. Pacing Clin Electrophysiol 1995;18(5 Pt 1): 1032–6.

16. Platt S, Furman S, Gross JN, et al. Transtelephonic monitoring for pacemaker follow-up 1981–1994. Pacing Clin Electrophysiol 1996;19:2089–98.

17. Sweesy MW, Erickson SL, Crago JA, et al. Analysis of the effectiveness of in-office and transtelephonic follow-up in terms of pacemaker system complications. Pacing Clin Electrophysiol 1994;17:2001–3.

18. Crossely GH, Chen J, Choucair W, et al. Clinical benefits of remote versus transtelephonic monitoring of implanted pacemakers. J Am Coll Cardiol 2009; 54:2012–9.

19. Varma N, Epstein AE, Irimpen A, et al, TRUST Investigators. Efficacy and safety of automatic remote monitoring for implantable cardioverter-defibrillator follow-up: the Lumos-T Safely Reduces Routine Office Device Follow-up (TRUST) trial. Circulation 2010;122:325–32.

20. Crossley GH, Boyle A, Vitense H, et al, CONNECT Investigators. The CONNECT (Clinical evaluation of remote notification to reduce time to clinical decision) trial. J Am Coll Cardiol 2011;57:1181–9.

21. Saxon LA, Hayes DL, Gilliam FR, et al. Long-term outcome after ICD and CRT implantation and influence of remote device follow-up: the ALTITUDE survival study. Circulation 2010;122:2359–67.

22. Wilkoff BL, Auricchio A, Brugada J, et al. HRS/EHRA Expert Consensus on the Monitoring of Cardiovascular Implantable Electronic Devices (CIEDs): description of techniques, indications, personnel, frequency and ethical considerations: developed in partnership with the Heart Rhythm Society (HRS) and the European Heart Rhythm Association (EHRA); and in collaboration with the American College of Cardiology (ACC), the American Heart Association (AHA), the European Society of Cardiology (ESC), the Heart Failure Association of ESC (HFA), and the Heart Failure Society of America (HFSA). Endorsed by the Heart Rhythm Society, the European Heart Rhythm Association (a registered branch of the ESC), the American College of Cardiology, the American Heart Association. Europace 2008;10:707–25.

23. Fryback DG, Thornbury JR. The efficacy of diagnostic imaging. Med Decis Making 1991;11(2):88–94.

Clinical Guidelines for Remote Monitoring

Sarah Bonnell, BS[a,b], Suneet Mittal, MD, FACC, FHRS[a,b,c],*

KEYWORDS

- Cardiac implantable electronic devices (CIEDs) • Guidelines • Remote monitoring

KEY POINTS

- Cardiac implantable electronic devices (CIEDs), which include implantable loop recorders, permanent pacemakers, implantable cardioverter-defibrillators, cardiac resynchronization therapy-permanent pacemakers, and cardiac resynchronization therapy-implantable cardioverter-defibrillators, are routinely used in clinical practice.
- The Heart Rhythm Society and European Heart Rhythm Association have previously published an expert consensus document that outlines the recommended frequency of CIED follow-up over the lifetime of the device.
- The advent of wireless technology has made it feasible to monitor CIED function and disease states (eg, atrial fibrillation, ventricular tachyarrhythmias, congestive heart failure) on a 24/7/365 basis.
- To date, no guidelines exist that provide recommendations on the optimal use of remote monitoring in clinical practice.

BACKGROUND

A variety of cardiac implantable electronic devices (CIEDs) are used routinely in clinical practice. These devices include implantable loop recorders (ILRs), permanent pacemakers (PPMs), implantable cardioverter-defibrillators (ICDs), cardiac resynchronization therapy (CRT)-PPMs, and CRT-ICDs. Following implantation, these devices require either in-office or remote follow-up. Herein the current guidelines for remote monitoring and follow-up of CIEDs are reviewed.

The Heart Rhythm Society and the European Heart Rhythm Association have identified 4 distinct goals for CIED monitoring (**Box 1**).[1] The first goal is to improve the patient's quality of life by optimizing device programming to ensure that they meet the patient's clinical needs. The second goal is to ensure proper assessment of device function (eg, battery longevity, lead integrity, etc). The third goal is to manage the patient's underlying disease through knowledge of underlying atrial and ventricular arrhythmias as well as indices that may portend an exacerbation of congestive heart failure. The fourth and final goal is to communicate effectively the retrieved information to the patient and all health care providers involved in the patient's medical care.

To meet these goals, information from CIEDs must be retrieved at regular intervals. Current recommendations advocate that all CIEDs be checked through direct patient contact within 72 hours of implant and again within 2 to 12 weeks after implant. Interestingly, a recent review of Medicare beneficiaries shows that only 42.4% of

Disclosures: S. Bonnell: None; and S. Mittal: Consultant to Ambucor.
[a] Arrhythmia Institute, Valley Health System, Columbia University College of Physicians and Surgeons, New York, NY, USA; [b] Arrhythmia Institute, Valley Health System, Columbia University College of Physicians and Surgeons, Ridgewood, NJ, USA; [c] Electrophysiology Laboratory, The Valley Hospital, 223 North Van Dien Avenue, Ridgewood, NJ 07450, USA
* Corresponding author. Electrophysiology Laboratory, The Valley Hospital, 223 North Van Dien Avenue, Ridgewood, NJ 07450.
E-mail address: mittsu@valleyhealth.com

Box 1
Goals of CIED monitoring

Patient related

- Optimize the patient's quality of life
- Optimize pacemaker/ICD system function to meet the patient's clinical requirements
- Identify patients at risk and initiate appropriate follow-up with field safety corrective action/safety alerts
- Triage non-CIED-related health problems and make appropriate referrals

CIED related

- Document appropriate CIED function
- Identify and correct abnormal CIED behavior
- Maximize pulse generator longevity while maintaining patient safety
- Identify CIEDs approaching end of battery life, to identify leads at risk of failure, and to organize CIED replacements in a nonemergent manner

Disease related

- Document the nature and frequency of arrhythmias over time and correlate with patient symptoms and determine the appropriateness of CIED response to these arrhythmias
- Document (when feasible) hemodynamic status, transthoracic impedance, patient activity, and other physiologic parameters over time as part of chronic disease monitoring in heart failure
- Monitor response to therapy

Communication

- Maintain a patient database
- Timely communication to the patient and relevant health care providers of CIED and disease-related information
- Provide technical expertise and education to colleagues, patients, and community

Abbreviations: CIED, cardiac implantable electronic device; ICD, implantable cardioverter-defibrillator.

Adapted from Wilkoff BL, Auricchio A, Brugada J, et al. HRS/EHRA expert consensus on the monitoring of cardiovascular implantable electronic devices (CIEDs): description of techniques, indications, personnel, frequency, and ethical considerations. Europace 2008;10:707–25; with permission.

---

resynchronization therapy – pacemaker (CRT-Ps), and cardiac resynchronization therapy – defibrillator (CRT-Ds) should generally be evaluated every 3 to 6 months. As one gets closer to the end of a battery's expected longevity, follow-up needs to be intensified, generally to every 1 to 3 months depending on the device and the patient's underlying rhythm. It is recommended that, at a minimum, an in-office evaluation be performed annually; all other follow-up evaluations can be performed either remotely or in-office (**Box 2**).[1,3]

REMOTE FOLLOW-UP

Although in-office visits for device check serve an important purpose (**Box 3**), technology has long been sought that can obviate routine in-office visits. Prospective studies have shown that patient compliance with the desired in-office follow-up schedule is low and that most in-office visits do not result in the need for any significant reprogramming.[4] The first foray into remote follow-up was the use of transtelephonic monitoring (TTM) to monitor PPM function. In this type of monitoring, the patient transmits data to their physician over a standard analog phone line. However, only limited information about battery longevity, presenting rhythm, and the adequacy of atrial and/or ventricular sensing and capture can be determined.

Box 2
Minimum frequency of CIED in-person or remote follow-up

Pacemakers/ICDs/CRTs

- Within 72 hours of CIED implantation (in-person)
- 2–12 weeks after implantation (in-person)
- Every 3–12 months pacemaker/CRT-P (in-person or remote)
- Every 3–6 months ICD/CRT-D (in-person or remote)
- Annually until battery depletion (in-person)
- Every 1–3 months at signs of battery depletion (in-person or remote)

Implantable loop recorder

- Every 1–6 months depending on patient symptoms and indication (in-person or remote)

Adapted from Wilkoff BL, Auricchio A, Brugada J, et al. HRS/EHRA expert consensus on the monitoring of cardiovascular implantable electronic devices (CIEDs): description of techniques, indications, personnel, frequency, and ethical considerations. Europace 2008;10:707–25; with permission.

---

eligible patients who underwent CIED implantation between 2005 and 2009 actually had an initial in-person evaluation within 2 to 12 weeks.[2] Subsequently, PPMs should be evaluated every 3 to 12 months, whereas ICDs, cardiac

---

Box 3
The pros and cons of remote monitoring and follow-up

In-office Visits	
Pros	Cons
Direct face-to-face contact	*Inefficient*
• Inspect device pocket	• Expense related to fuel, parking, tolls, taking off from work
• Convey recent health history, including change in medications	• Most commonly no intervention is required
• Assurance that information has been retrieved and interpreted	

Over time, CIEDs became capable of storing more diagnostic information. For example, devices routinely track battery longevity, trends in P-wave and R-wave amplitude, lead impedance, and information on pacing percentage. In addition, information on arrhythmias such as atrial fibrillation and ventricular tachycardia/fibrillation is stored. The availability to retrieve and adjudicate stored electrograms has facilitated the ability of the physician to target therapy to the individual patient. Finally, there are active attempts to track indices (eg, weight, blood pressure, transthoracic impedance) that may identify patients at impending risk for developing an exacerbation of congestive heart failure. These diagnostic data cannot be retrieved using TTM. Rather, remote follow-up systems were developed that could, with the exception of inhibiting pacing or performing manual threshold checks, replicate an in-office device interrogation. Initially, similar to TTM, patient involvement was required. The patient needed to place a wand over their implanted device and initiate an interrogation, which could then be transmitted over an analog phone line to a central web-based workstation for physician review. Today, all ILRs, PPMs, CRT-Ps, and CRT-Ds can all be followed remotely in this manner. Studies performed to date have demonstrated that remote follow-up systems can reduce the burden of in-office visits (which tend to be very resource intensive) and increase patient satisfaction.[4–6]

REMOTE MONITORING

More recently, devices have become capable of transmitting the data wirelessly over a cellular network, thus eliminating the need for patient involvement in the data transmission process. This elimination of patient involvement has ushered in the process of remote monitoring, in which the patient and physician are tethered to each other on a 24/7/265 basis. Critical alerts can be transmitted to physicians immediately as opposed to the time of the next patient-initiated transmission. Although previously available commercially,[7] wireless ILRs are currently not being marketed. However, most PPMs and all ICDs and CRT-Ds being implanted today are capable of wireless remote monitoring. In contrast to in-office device checks, there are several inherent pros and cons to remote monitoring and follow-up (**Box 4**).

The TRUST trial compared the safety and efficacy of remote monitoring to quarterly in-office evaluation in a cohort of non-pacemaker-dependent patients following single-chamber or dual-chamber ICD implantation. Home monitoring reduced the need for in-office evaluations by 45% without adversely affecting morbidity. In addition, home monitoring reduced the time to evaluation for arrhythmic events (atrial fibrillation, supraventricular tachycardia, ventricular tachycardia, and fibrillation) to less than 2 days.[8] The same was true for the detection of problems with the ICD leads or generator.[9] More recently, the ECOST trial further extended the value of remote monitoring in ICD patients.[10] In this trial of 433 ICD patients, 212 patients underwent in-office device evaluation every 6 months. The other 221 patients underwent in-office evaluation yearly unless remote monitoring reported an ICD dysfunction or clinical event requiring an in-office visit. Over a mean follow-up

---

Box 4
The pros and cons of in-office device checks

Remote Evaluation	
Pros	Cons
Remote follow-up	*Patient participation necessary*
• Save time and expense related to proceeding with an in-office check	• Connect system
	• Transmit information (non-wireless systems)
Remote monitoring	
• Early notification of critical information	*"Faith based"*
	• Is information being retrieved, interpreted, and communicated?

of 24.2 months, both groups experienced a similar incidence of a major adverse event (death from any cause as well as any cardiovascular-related, procedure-related, or device-related major adverse events). However, the remote monitoring group was significantly less likely to receive an inappropriate or appropriate ICD shock.

Despite these promising data, to date there are no guidelines that address the appropriate use of remote monitoring in clinical practice. Thus, it is not entirely surprising that up to one-third of patients with a device capable of remote monitoring are not being enrolled into a remote monitoring program; of enrolled patients, only a small number are actually transmitting data on a quarterly basis.[11] Although guidelines are clearly needed, the following challenges should be adequately recognized and addressed for any proposed guidelines to be practical.

CHALLENGES TO REMOTE MONITORING AND FOLLOW-UP

Neither remote follow-up nor remote monitoring is possible unless the patient understands the importance of these "nonoffice" virtual interactions for the management of their devices and underlying disease conditions. The patient then has to consent to being enrolled into a remote program, connect the equipment once it arrives at their home, and complete the initial "hand check" transmission. Therefore, an established protocol for patient education is a key factor in building a solid foundation of trust with the patient toward remote monitoring and follow-up and ensuring sustained compliance (**Fig. 1**).[11]

A representative of industry, allied health professional, or physician can initiate the education process during the initial consultation, during the immediate perioperative or postoperative period, or at the first postimplant office visit. During this educational process, as per a current Heart Rhythm Society/European Heart Rhythm Association consensus document, a "care agreement" with a patient is developed.[1] This agreement fosters a mutual understanding of the type of care than can be expected and the roles and responsibilities of all providers involved in the care of the patient with a CEID. Especially important is a review of a clinic's protocols that identify the time it takes to respond to critical data and the mechanism by which data are communicated to the patient and his/her other health care providers. A consensus on the optimal method for patient education and minimum requirements for clinic protocols is necessary.

In the authors' practice, they have identified 5 major factors that prevent them from universally having patients actively followed in a remote monitoring and follow-up program (**Fig. 2**). The single biggest barrier is technology. Many, especially older, patients fear that they will not be able to connect the remote monitoring system correctly once it arrives to their home. The need to connect it to an analog phone line has been a particularly important barrier. Some patients do not take the

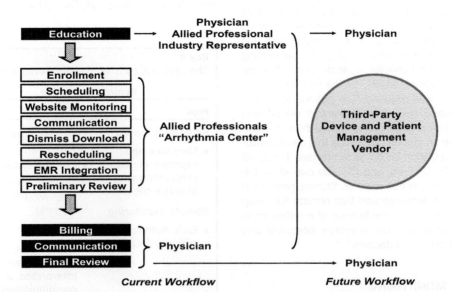

Fig. 1. The workflow inherent to running a successful remote monitoring and follow-up program. (*From* Movsowitz C, Mittal S. Remote patient management using implanted devices. J Interv Card Electrophysiol 2011;31: 81–90; with permission.)

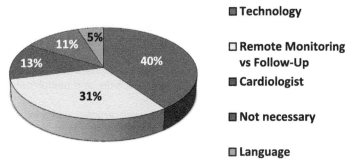

Fig. 2. The 5 major barriers to patient enrollment into a remote monitoring and follow-up program. See text for discussion.

initiative of "splitting" their analog phone line to connect their remote monitoring system; for others, the use of a cable or VoIP (voice over Internet protocols) telephone system precludes seamless operation of the remote systems. The ideal system is the Biotronik Home Monitoring system; this only requires that the patient connect the unit into a power outlet. Data transmission then occurs seamlessly over a Global System for Mobile communications–based cellular network. Although other vendors also offer a Global System for Mobile communications–based remote system, the patient needs to pay the monthly charge for cellular service; this is something most patients are unwilling to accept, especially older patients on fixed incomes.

The second most important barrier is the inability of patients to grasp the difference between remote monitoring and remote follow-up. The latter can obviate some in-office visits but cannot completely eliminate them because the authors recommend an annual in-office visit for all CIED patients. Many patients welcome the increased convenience of remote follow-up; others dislike the concept, as they prefer face-to-face contact with their physician. Before guidelines for remote monitoring can be developed, patients will need to understand the value to continuous surveillance to optimize device and disease management. To date, this has been difficult to accomplish in clinical practice. Nonetheless, device/lead integrity data, atrial and ventricular arrhythmias, and other information stored within the device should be accessed more than the traditional quarterly or bi-annual basis to monitor the patient's progress.

The next important issue is to understand the role and belief of the referring cardiologist. In 13% of patients, the cardiologists ask to take responsibility for remote monitoring and/or follow-up. Disappointingly, in another 11% of patients, the referring cardiologist specifically discourages

the patient from remote monitoring and follow-up, typically citing the absence of clinical guidelines. Finally, in a small number of patients, a language barrier precludes them from understanding the available literature from vendors on remote systems, because there is very little information available in a language other than English.

Guidelines on remote monitoring must address the optimal infrastructure necessary to handle the large volume of incoming data emanating from wireless CIEDs. In addition, data accumulate through interaction of CIED patients with health care personnel in settings such as the emergency room, operating room, radiology suite, and inpatient hospital floors (Fig. 3). The data must be reviewed to ensure that all device/lead advisories

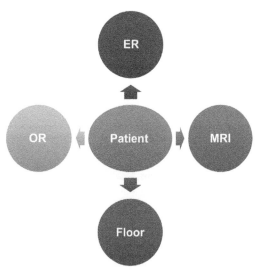

Fig. 3. Sites of encounters between the CIED patient and health care personnel. The ideal remote monitoring infrastructure should permit centralization of all data emanating from CIED device-patient encounters with health care personnel in the emergency room (ER), operating room (OR), radiology suite (eg, MRI suite), and in-hospital floor locations.

are accounted for, pacing algorithms have been optimized to minimize the degree of right ventricular pacing and maximize the degree of biventricular pacing, atrial high rate episodes are appropriately adjudicated and a plan for management (eg, anticoagulation) defined, devices programmed to minimize inappropriate and appropriate ICD shocks, and signs of impending heart failure identified. In addition, data must be accounted for on a 24/7/365 basis to ensure that information is not missed that could adversely affect a patient's clinical outcome, a major barrier to overcome, which contributes to a concern about the legal liability inherent to managing these data.

One method for handling the data emanating from remote monitoring and follow-up systems is to delegate the responsibility to a dedicated group who can notify individual clinics of important notifications. The utility of this type of approach was recently evaluated in the MoniC study.[12] In this prospective, multicenter study, a centralized monitoring center was responsible for monitoring remote patient data for 9 satellite device clinics. A trained telemonitoring nurse categorized all notifications into "red," "yellow," and "green" categories, representing urgent/highly important data, potentially important data, or data for which immediate notification is not necessary, respectively. Notifications triggered interventions such as a phone call to the patient, a medication change, and/or device reprogramming. The MoniC study concluded that this approach was a highly reliable, safe, and useful tool for providing remote care.

Future remote monitoring guidelines will need to recognize that many practices will be unable to absorb the administrative and personnel costs inherent to the operation of a large virtual clinic in parallel to standard in-office sessions. In keeping with the findings of the MoniC study, the authors agree with the use of "neutral" third-party providers to handle the growing need to manage data within a practice that manages CIED patients (see **Fig. 1**). The authors have incorporated the Ambucor Health Solutions CardioView Dx Suite, which supports all ambulatory external electrocardiogram monitoring modalities (Holter, event monitoring, mobile ambulatory cardiovascular [real-time] telemetry monitoring), ambulatory 24-hour blood pressure monitoring, and monitoring of all implantable devices (**Fig. 4**). The data are maintained on the CardioFile database, which is maintained on the "cloud" (**Fig. 5**), can be accessed from any Internet-enabled personal computer in the world, and is capable of communicating to a

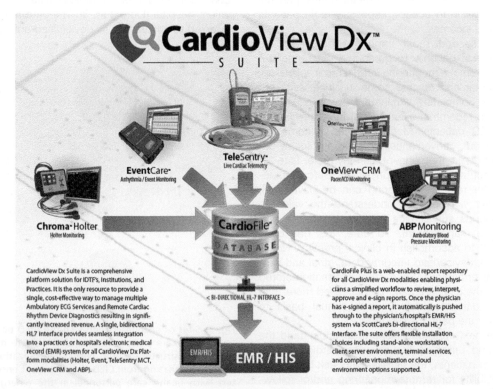

Fig. 4. The CardioView Dx suite. See text for discussion. (*From* Mittal S, Steinberg JS. Remote patient monitoring in cardiology: a case-based guide. New York: Demos Medical; 2012; with permission.)

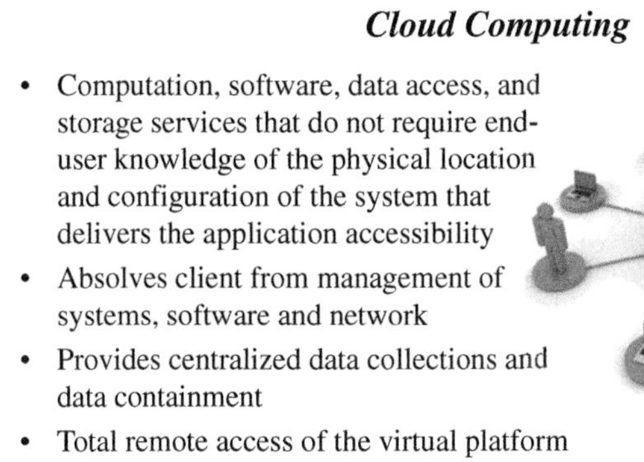

Cloud Computing

- Computation, software, data access, and storage services that do not require end-user knowledge of the physical location and configuration of the system that delivers the application accessibility
- Absolves client from management of systems, software and network
- Provides centralized data collections and data containment
- Total remote access of the virtual platform

Fig. 5. The principles and advantages of cloud computing. (*From* Mittal S, Steinberg JS. Remote patient monitoring in cardiology: a case-based guide. New York: Demos Medical; 2012; with permission.)

practice/hospital electronic medical record system via a bi-directional HL-7 interface. The OneView CRM platform (**Fig. 6**) can handle data from all major device manufacturers from device implantation through the life of the device (both in-office and remote). Importantly, all types of data are collected (routine device assessment, arrhythmia detection, heart failure evaluation), communication provided to patients and providers, and assistance provided to ensure complete capture of billing data, all on a 24/7/365 basis.[13]

A final important issue relates to reimbursement. To facilitate the adoption of remote follow-up, the United States Center for Medicare and Medicaid Services provides reimbursement on a monthly basis for ILRs and on a quarterly basis for PPMs, CRT-Ps, ICDs, and CRT-Ds, in line with current recommendations for minimum CIED monitoring

(see **Box 1**). However, outside the United States, the reimbursement policy is less well defined, which influences adoption of this technology.[14] A recent European Heart Rhythm Association survey (involving 14 European centers and 1 in Tunisia) reported a lack of reimbursement in 82% of countries; not surprisingly, 40% of centers reported using remote monitoring on a "frequent" basis.[15] TARIFF, an ongoing Italian study, is designed to compare direct and indirect costs and benefits of in-office versus remote monitoring and follow-up of ICD and CRT-D patients.[16] Data on quality of life, hospitalizations, and ambulatory visits will be collected. Ultimately, the study intends to study the cost and the value of remote monitoring of health care services, to help the Italian medical system make decisions regarding their reimbursement and supply to the hospitals.

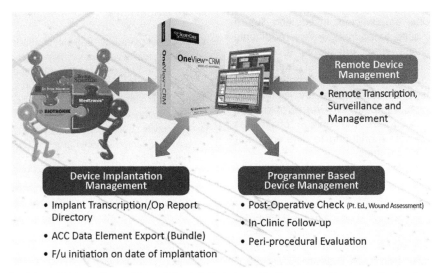

Fig. 6. The OneView CRM platform. (*From* Mittal S, Steinberg JS. Remote patient monitoring in cardiology: a case-based guide. New York: Demos Medical; 2012; with permission.)

> **Box 5**
> **Areas for future research**
>
> 1. What is the sensitivity and specificity of data obtained from CIEDs under various specific conditions?
> 2. What is the time interval between CIED-based detection of an abnormality and measures to be taken by the responsible physician or the patient?
> 3. Although remote monitoring is intended to reduce the need for some face-to-face scheduled clinic visits, what is its impact on various outcome parameters, such as quality of life, adverse events, even mortality, etc?
> 4. With increasing number of patients with CIEDs, what is the impact on physician and technician working load?
> 5. What is the cost-effectiveness ratio of such systems?
> 6. What are the potential, not yet identified problems with regard to patient data protection, and what are the potential differences of these problems with various national and international legal systems (with data stored outside one's own country)?
>
> *Adapted from* Dubner S, Auricchio A, Steinberg JS, et al. ISHNE/EHRA expert consensus on remote monitoring of cardiovascular implantable electronic devices (CIEDs). Europace 2012;14:278–93; with permission.

SUMMARY

The technology now exists to permit routine remote monitoring and follow-up of CIED patients. In this article, the existing challenges that need to be overcome are outlined. In addition, future research will need to address several additional important unanswered questions (**Box 5**).[17] Currently, clinical guidelines that outline the optimal approach to incorporating remote technology into routine clinical practice are lacking. To have a meaningful impact, any set of guidelines will need to recognize the unique challenges imposed by remote monitoring to different practices in different countries.

REFERENCES

1. Wilkoff BL, Auricchio A, Brugada J, et al. HRS/EHRA expert consensus on the monitoring of cardiovascular implantable electronic devices (CIEDs): description of techniques, indications, personnel, frequency, and ethical considerations. Europace 2008;10:707–25.

2. Al-Khatib SM, Mi X, Wilkoff BL, et al. Follow-up of patients with new cardiovascular implantable electronic devices: are experts' recommendations implemented in routine clinical practice? Circ Arrhythm Electrophysiol 2013. http://dx.doi.org/10.1161/CIRCEP.112.974337.

3. Tracy CM, Epstein AE, Darbar D, et al. 2012 ACCF/AHA/HRS focused update of the 2008 guidelines for device-based therapy of cardiac rhythm abnormalities. J Am Coll Cardiol 2012;60:1297–313.

4. Udo EO, van Hemel NM, Zuithoff NP, et al. Pacemaker follow-up: are the latest guidelines in line with modern pacemaker practice? Europace 2013. http://dx.doi.org/10.1093/europace/eus310.

5. Burri H, Senouf D. Remote monitoring and follow-up of pacemakers and implantable cardioverter defibrillators. Europace 2009;11:701–9.

6. Boriani G, Auricchio A, Klersy C, et al. Healthcare personnel resource burden related to in-clinic follow-up of cardiovascular implantable electronic devices: a European Heart Rhythm Association and Eucomed joint survey. Europace 2011;13:1166–73.

7. Paruchuri V, Adhaduk M, Garikipati NV, et al. Clinical utility of a novel wireless implantable loop recorder in the evaluation of patients with unexplained syncope. Heart Rhythm 2011;8:858–63.

8. Varma N, Epstein A, Irimpen A, et al. The lumos-T safety routine efficacy and safety of automatic remote monitoring for implantable cardioverter defibrillator follow-up. The lumos-T safely reduces routine office device follow-up (TRUST) trial. Circulation 2010;122:325–32.

9. Varma N, Michalski J, Epstein AE, et al. Automatic remote monitoring of implantable cardioverter-defibrillator lead and generator performance: the lumos-T safely reduces routine office device follow-up (TRUST) trial. Circ Arrhythm Electrophysiol 2010;3:428–36.

10. Guedon-Moreau L, Lacroix D, Sadoul N, et al, ECOST trial investigators. A randomized study of remote follow-up of implantable cardioverter defibrillators: safety and efficacy report of the ECOST trial. Eur Heart J 2013. http://dx.doi.org/10.1093/eurheartj/ehs425.

11. Movsowitz C, Mittal S. Remote patient management using implanted devices. J Interv Card Electrophysiol 2011;31:81–90.

12. Vogtmann T, Stiller S, Marek A, et al. Workload and usefulness of daily, centralized home monitoring for patients treated with CIEDs: results of the MoniC (Model Project Monitor Centre) prospective multicenter study. Europace 2012. http://dx.doi.org/10.1093/europace/eus252.

13. Mittal S, Steinberg JS, editors. Remote patient monitoring in cardiology: a case-based guide. 1st edition. New York: Demos Medical; 2012.

14. Varma N, Ricci RP. Telemedicine and cardiac implants: what is the benefit? Eur Heart J 2013. http://dx.doi.org/10.1093/eurheartj/ehs388.

15. Halimi F, Canti F, on behalf of the European Heart Rhythm Association (EHRA) Scientific Initiatives Committee (SIC). Remote monitoring for active cardiovascular implantable electronic devices: a European survey. Europace 2010;12:1778–80.

16. Ricci RP, D'Onofrio A, Padeletti L, et al. Rationale and design of the health economics evaluation registry for remote follow-up: TARIFF. Europace 2012; 14:1661–5.

17. Dubner S, Auricchio A, Steinberg JS, et al. ISHNE/ EHRA expert consensus on remote monitoring of cardiovascular implantable electronic devices (CIEDs). Europace 2012;14:278–93.

Device Monitoring

Casey Cable, MD, Fred M. Kusumoto, MD*

KEYWORDS

- Pacemaker • Cardiac defibrillatior • Monitoring

KEY POINTS

- Routine remote monitoring of implanted cardiac devices offers several advantages, including arrhythmia detection, assessment of ablation procedure efficacy, and monitoring of leads and devices for the early identification of potential hardware problems.
- Several well-done clinical trials, such as ASSERT, EVOLVO, and PREFER, have demonstrated the success of using remote monitoring technologies to identify patient-related and device-related problems.
- The significant increase in data being delivered to busy cardiac device clinics for analysis will have important ramifications on physician-nurse workflow and resource utilization in the future and these needs will have to be addressed and optimized to make full use of such technologies.

Implanted devices, such as pacemakers and cardiac defibrillators (ICDs), have become an established treatment for patients with symptomatic bradycardia or those who are at risk for sudden cardiac death. In the last decade, implantable loop recorders have emerged as a diagnostic tool for the evaluation of patients with intermittent symptoms that may be due to arrhythmias, and cardiac resynchronization therapy is now an essential therapy for selected patients with heart failure. It is currently estimated that worldwide approximately 1 million pacemakers and 300,000 ICDs are implanted every year.[1] Although clinicians often focus on the initial device implant, an equally and perhaps more important aspect of device therapy is continuous evaluation of the patient and device after implant. For example, several multicenter studies have demonstrated that programming devices to minimize right ventricular–only pacing is important for reducing episodes of heart failure.[2,3]

The large number of implanted cardiac devices has important ramifications for health care costs and resource utilization. The traditional model of in-person follow-up at a medical clinic requires significant investment in manpower and technology and indirect costs due to lost productivity from the patient with the implanted device. Early identification of device problems such as lead failures or accelerated battery depletion is essential for maximizing the benefits of device therapy. For example, in the traditionally accepted model of defibrillator evaluations every 6 months, if a lead were to fail just after an in-office visit, the patient would be exposed to risk of ventricular arrhythmias with inadequate treatment for a prolonged period of time.

The potential problems with in-office device follow-up have been understood for many years and the first method for trying to improve the continuity of device follow-up was transtelephonic monitoring (TTM). Introduced in the 1970s, with rudimentary monitoring capabilities, the initial goal of TTM was to monitor battery life and also provide a limited analysis of underlying rhythm and ventricular capture. In today's generation of devices, methods for remote monitoring of device function have replaced TTM. Remote monitoring provides a more complete analysis of device function and also allows transmission of large amounts of data that has been gathered by the device.

Disclosures: The authors have nothing to disclose.
Electrophysiology and Pacing Service, Division of Cardiovascular disease, Department of Medicine, 4500 San Pablo Avenue, Jacksonville, FL 32224, USA
* Corresponding author.
E-mail address: Kusumoto.fred@mayo.edu

Depending on the system, remote monitoring can provide almost instant identification of deterioration in clinical status or abnormalities in device function. Remote monitoring is particularly useful for identification and monitoring of arrhythmias and for timely identification of abnormal device function.

EARLY DETECTION OF PROBLEMS

Remote monitoring capabilities were first developed in ICDs, and early on investigators recognized the potential of remote monitoring for timely identification of problems. In the first proof-of-concept study of remote monitoring, 59 patients with ICDs were asked to send 2 transmissions, at least 7 days apart, via standard phone line to a secure server.[4] Problems with transmission of information occurred about 10% of the time. Importantly, even with this minimal transmission of information, several clinical problems were identified, including atrial undersensing, T-wave undersensing, and new onset atrial fibrillation.

Since this first cohort study, there have been 7 randomized trials that compared follow-up with remote monitoring and traditional follow-up with in-office visits only (**Table 1**). Five of the 7 trials studied remote monitoring in patients with ICDs

Table 1
Randomized studies on remote monitoring

Trial (Sponsor)	Number (Initially Enrolled)	Follow-up	Findings
Pacemaker			
PREFER (Medtronic)	897 (980)	12 mo	Remote monitoring reduced the time for identifying "actionable events" from 8 mo to 6 mo
COMPAS (Biotronik)	494 (538)	18 mo	Remote monitoring was a safe alternative to conventional care and significantly lowered the number of ambulatory visits
ICD			
TRUST (Biotronik)	908 (1339)	15 mo	Remote monitoring reduced the time for arrhythmia identification, from 36 d to less than 2 d
EVATEL (French Department of Health)	1434 (1501)	12 mo	No difference in remote follow-up vs office visit follow-up in preventing major clinic adverse event
ECOST (Biotronik)	433	24 mo	Remote monitoring significantly lowered the number of appropriate and inappropriate shocks delivered
ICD/CRT-D			
CONNECT (Medtronic)	1980 (1997)	15 mo	Remote monitoring reduced the time from clinical event to clinical decision from 22 d to 5 d
EVOLVO (Medtronic)	200	16 mo	Identification of worsening heart failure by remote monitoring was associated with rapid assessment of patient status (less than 2 d) with a 35% decrease in emergency department or urgent in-office evaluation

Abbreviations: CRT, cardiac resynchronization therapy; ECOST, Benefits of Implantable Defibrillator Follow-up Using Remote Monitoring; EVOLVO, Evolution of Management Strategies of Heart Failure Patients with Implantable Defibrillators.
Data from Refs.[5–7,12,15,36,37]

and 2 trials evaluated remote monitoring in patients with pacemakers. One of the common findings in all of the trials has been early identification of clinical problems. For example, in the Clinical Evaluation of Remote Monitoring to Reduce Time to Clinical Decision (CONNECT) study, 1997 patients were randomized to follow-up with or without remote monitoring.[5] During a follow-up of 15 months, remote monitoring reduced the time from clinical event to clinical decision from 22 days to 5 days. Atrial arrhythmias longer than 12 hours or atrial arrhythmias associated with a rapid ventricular rate accounted for 90% of the clinical events. Similarly, in the Lumos T Safely Reduces Routine Office Device Follow-up Trial (TRUST), remote monitoring reduced the time for arrhythmia identification from 36 days to less than 2 days.[6] In addition, identification of "actionable events" (events that required programming changes, change in medication) was 50% higher in the remote monitoring group. In contrast to the CONNECT study, in TRUST, 75% of the arrhythmias detected by remote monitoring were ventricular tachycardia or ventricular fibrillation, and only 25% were atrial arrhythmias.

The clinical benefit of remote monitoring will depend on how monitoring is performed, patient characteristics, and device type. For example, in one study that evaluated patients with pacemakers (Pacemaker Remote Follow-up Evaluation and Review [PREFER] study), remote monitoring reduced the time for identifying "actionable events" from 8 months to 6 months, in part because the study design performed remote monitoring every 2 months.[7] The extremely rapid identification of abnormal arrhythmias in the TRUST study was in part caused by a remote monitoring system that allows almost continuous transfer of data from the ICD to a central server without requiring the patient to perform any specific tasks.[6] It is obvious then that remote monitoring is often used interchangeably to describe remote episodic interrogation or frequent automatic transmission of data from the device to a centralized server. The actual "mechanics" of remote monitoring also have important workflow ramifications (**Fig. 1**). In a recent workflow analysis at a busy device clinic, although remote monitoring was associated with a significant decrease in time spent on analysis when compared with traditional in-clinic visits (27.7 minutes to 11.5 minutes), almost 50% of scheduled transmissions were missed due to patient compliance.[8] Automated remote monitoring seems to be more reliable but not foolproof. In TRUST, transmission reliability was greater than 90%.[9]

The clinical benefit of remote monitoring for early identification of an arrhythmia will depend on the likelihood of arrhythmia in a given patient. In the Asymptomatic Atrial Fibrillation and Stroke Evaluation in Pacemaker Patients and the Atrial Fibrillation Reduction Atrial Pacing Trial (ASSERT), 2580 patients without a prior history of atrial fibrillation had pacemakers or ICDs implanted.[10] After 2.5 years of follow-up, approximately 10% of patients had device-detected atrial fibrillation. In contrast, in an analysis of 4 studies of patients with heart failure and cardiac resynchronization devices, atrial fibrillation was identified in 33% of patients.[11] Although not formally studied, it is likely that the absolute benefit of remote monitoring will be higher in sicker patients with more dynamic changes in their cardiovascular status.

Generally, remote monitoring has focused on early identification of atrial and ventricular tachyarrhythmias. As devices become more sophisticated, remote monitoring may be useful for early identification of problems not specifically related to arrhythmias. In the recently published Evolution of Management Strategies of Heart Failure Patients with Implantable Defibrillators study, 315 alerts were identified in 99 patients followed by remote monitoring.[12] In this study, 87% of the alerts were due to possible worsening of heart failure identified by changes in thoracic impedance. Identification of worsening heart failure by remote monitoring was associated with rapid assessment of patient status (less than 2 days) by telephone and after 16 months of follow-up was associated with a 35% decrease in emergency department or urgent in-office evaluation. Another study using the same technology, the Randomized Clinical Evaluation of Wireless Fluid Monitoring and Remote ICD Management using Optivol (CONNECT-OptiVol) study, is currently being performed to evaluate whether remote monitoring will prolong the time to first hospitalization for heart failure.[13]

In addition to identifying patient-related clinical problems, such as arrhythmias or worsening heart failure, an important use of remote monitoring is early identification of device-related problems. In the TRUST trial, 43 system-related alerts occurred in 32 of the 908 patients followed over a 15-month follow-up period.[14] In 20 patients, possible ineffectiveness of the maximum device output (25 J) was identified. Twelve of these patients (60%) had "actionable events," such as changes in programming, initiation of an antiarrhythmic medication, or lead revision. Possible lead problems were identified in 13 patients, and of these, 5 (29%) had actionable events such as lead revision or a programming change. More than 60% of the device failure–related alerts were identified within 24 hours of occurrence. Early identification of hardware

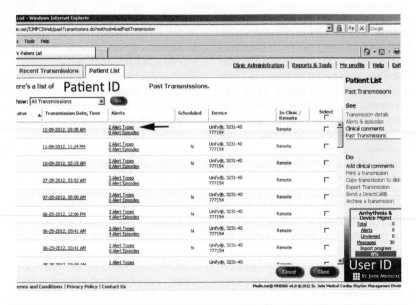

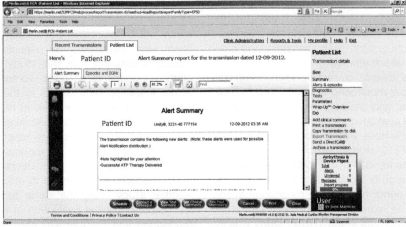

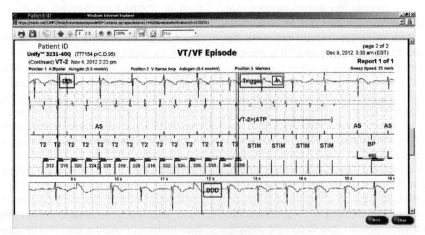

Fig. 1. Example of an alert from remote monitoring. (*top*) Initial Windows screen for a patient with an alert from a remote monitoring system (*arrow*). Clicking on the alert event will lead to a summary screen of the alert (*middle screen*). The user can scroll down the report to evaluate the electrograms. In this case, the patient had an episode of ventricular tachycardia; notice the relationship between atrial and ventricular EGMs. The patient receives anti-tachycardia pacing and the tachycardia was terminated. The device nurse called the patient the next day after the alert and found out the patient was completely asymptomatic.

problems can result in important clinical benefits. In the Benefits of Implantable Defibrillator Follow-up Using Remote Monitoring Trial, device-related problems were identified in 5.7% and 6.9% of the remote monitoring and control groups, respectively.[15] However, lead dysfunction without an inappropriate shock was much more common in the remote monitoring group (2.4% vs 0.5%). The likelihood of device-related problems identified by remote monitoring in patients with pacemakers is probably less than for patients with ICDs. In the PREFER trial, hardware problems accounted for less than 5% of all of the alerts.[7]

Another emerging use for remote monitoring is for facilitating early discharge of selected patients after implantation of a new ICD. In one study, 71 patients who underwent uncomplicated implantation of an ICD were randomized to same-day discharge with remote follow-up or traditional overnight observation.[16] In the 37 patients who were discharged after 4 hours, no changes in lead parameters were identified by remote monitoring in during the 24 hours after implant. Remote monitoring in the period just after initial implantation may be extremely useful, because this is the period in which lead malfunction caused by lead dislodgement is most likely to occur.

MONITORING FOR SPECIFIC ARRHYTHMIAS

Identification of arrhythmias is one of the most important functions of remote monitoring. Arrhythmias identified by a device may have important prognostic information. The type of arrhythmia detected by the device will depend on the clinical characteristics of the patient. Although not specifically designed to evaluate remote monitoring, as mentioned earlier, in ASSERT 10% of patients had subclinical atrial fibrillation identified by device interrogation.[10] Importantly, in this cohort, patients with atrial fibrillation identified by the device had a 6-fold increase in the likelihood of developing symptomatic atrial fibrillation and a 2.5-fold increase in risk of stroke or thromboembolism. Currently, it is not known whether anticoagulation therapy is beneficial in all patients with device-detected atrial fibrillation, but it is reasonable to consider anticoagulation in those patients with significant risk factors for stroke.

In addition to providing information on risk of thromboembolic events, remote monitoring of arrhythmias may have a use for evaluating efficacy of pharmacologic or nonpharmacologic therapy. More than 2 decades ago, the landmark Cardiac Arrhythmia Suppression Trial demonstrated that suppression of ventricular arrhythmias by antiarrhythmic drugs was associated with a higher mortality than placebo.[17] This critical finding helped accelerate the development of ICDs as the first-line therapy for those patients at highest risk for sudden cardiac death. Although ICDs provide an important "safety net" for the treatment of ventricular arrhythmias, adjunctive antiarrhythmic drug treatment is extremely useful in selected patients for reducing shocks. In the same era as the Cardiac Arrhythmia Suppression Trial, it was also noted that suppression of ventricular arrhythmias by 24-hour ambulatory electrocardiographic monitoring was equivalent to electrophysiologic testing, which was the "gold standard" at the time for evaluating antiarrhythmic drug efficacy.[18] Since then, sotalol and amiodarone have been found to reduce the requirement for ICD therapy.[19,20] More recently, newer antiarrhythmic medications such as dofetilide and azimilide have been shown to suppress ventricular arrhythmias in patients with ICDs, which reduced utilization of health care resources such as emergency room visits and hospitalization.[21,22] Although no studies are available, it is likely that remote monitoring of ventricular arrhythmia burden may be beneficial for continuous evaluation of the effectiveness of drug therapy. Similarly, remote monitoring may also be useful for guiding the effectiveness of nonpharmacologic therapy. For a similar purpose, several studies have evaluated the efficacy of ablation for atrial fibrillation with the use of implantable loop recorders.[23,24] The value of remote monitoring for following a patient with atrial fibrillation is shown in **Fig. 2**.

Evaluation of stored electrograms obtained during any saved episode is essential. **Fig. 3** is from a patient referred for recurrent "ventricular tachycardia." Notice that the ventriculoatrial interval during ventricular pacing is significantly shorter than during tachycardia. The bottom panel shows the tachycardia initiating with an atrial signal. This combination of findings suggests atrioventricular node reentrant tachycardia that was confirmed at electrophysiology study. The patient underwent successful slow pathway modification with subsequent elimination of his episodes of rapid heart rate requiring device therapy.

HARDWARE PROBLEMS AND RECALLS

Since the inception of implantable cardiac devices more than 50 years ago, there have been certain lead designs with higher than expected failure rates that were identified only after the lead became commercially available and had been implanted in large numbers. Given the harshness of the environment that the lead must function in, it is not surprising that certain lead designs are

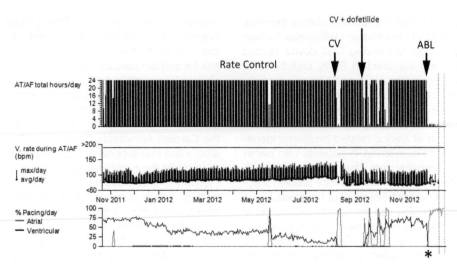

Fig. 2. Patient with persistent atrial fibrillation. Initially, the patient underwent attempts at rate control. Notice that even as β-blockers were increased, there was no effect on the ventricular rate, and actually the percentage of ventricular pacing decreased. Because the patient continued to be symptomatic, a simple cardioversion was performed but the patient had return to persistent atrial fibrillation. Cardioversion was repeated, this time with initiation of dofetilide. Initially the patient had paroxysmal atrial fibrillation, but unfortunately, after several weeks persistent atrial fibrillation developed. During this period the patient had more aggressive rate control as evidenced by the lower average heart rates and increased ventricular pacing. The patient underwent catheter ablation in early December and has now remained in sinus rhythm for the past 6 weeks with improvement in symptoms. Notice that in sinus rhythm, the patient has an increase in atrial pacing and elimination of ventricular pacing (*asterisk*). Remote monitoring allows assessment of rate control and ventricular pacing, and also whether sinus rhythm is maintained. This method of follow-up is particularly useful for patients who have a difficult time coming to the pacemaker clinic. ABL, ablation; AT/AF, atrial tachycardia/atrial fibrillation; CV, cardioversion.

found to be problematic after release. In the early 1990s, leads manufactured with a specific polyurethane (Pellethane 80A) were found to be susceptible to insulation problems and a 20% failure rate at 6 years.[25] Similarly, some first-generation ICD leads that used the same type of polyurethane were associated with a 40% failure rate at 7 years.[26] Although manufacturers have invested significant effort in developing more reliable leads, lead failures will continue to occur in the future. Already, remote monitoring has been identified as an important tool for early identification and management of patients who have leads with higher than expected failure rates.

In October 2007 Medtronic recalled the Sprint Fidelis leads as a Food and Drug Administration (FDA) class I recall (**Table 2** lists the recalls), which were initially introduced to the market in 2004. The FDA uses a classification system as an estimate of the risk when a manufacturer is trying to withdraw a product from the market. A class I recall is used to describe a product whereby there is a "reasonable probability" that exposure will cause "serious adverse health consequences or death." A class II recall is issued when the product may cause "temporary or reversible adverse health consequences" or the "probability of severe health

consequences is remote." A class III recall is one in which the manufacturer is trying to remove a product from the market but the product is "not likely to cause adverse health consequences." The recall for the Fidelis lead was due to increased risk of lead fracture after a small initial aftermarket study in 2007 revealed an increased failure rate of 1.1% at 2 years of implantation.[27] Medtronic confirmed these results with a follow-up analysis that found a 2.4% fracture rate at 30 months in October 2007. Subsequent studies continued to confirm increased lead failure rates at 3.75% annually.[28] Although there is some controversy in the rate of lead failure over time, there is no question that older leads are more susceptible to failure. In response to the high failure rate, Medtronic developed an algorithm using 3 components (impedance monitoring and 2 noise algorithms) and an automatic programming response that could be used to identify frank or impending lead failure quickly. The impedance component uses daily impedance measurements and compares maximal and average measurements over a weekly average to provide patient specificity. For example, if the average is less than 700 Ω, the threshold is 1000 Ω, but if the average is 700 Ω to 1100 Ω, the threshold is 1500 Ω. The first

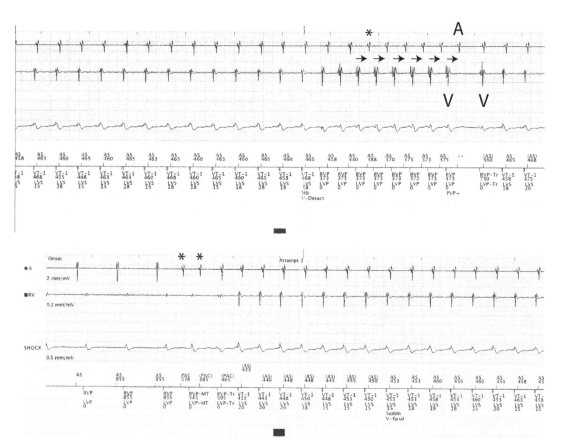

Fig. 3. EGMs saved from an event in a patient referred for ventricular tachycardia. (*top panel*) During tachycardia, the patient has a 1:1 relationship between atrial and ventricular events that can be observed in any supraventricular tachycardia (atrial tachycardia, tachycardia arising from the junction, accessory pathway mediated tachycardia) or ventricular tachycardia. Closer inspection of the atrial and ventricular signals demonstrates a very short V-A interval. With ventricular pacing, the first atrial signal that is entrained (*asterisk*) is associated with a much longer V-A interval, thus making the tachycardia much less likely to represent ventricular tachycardia or accessory pathway-mediated tachycardia. The patient has a V-A-V response on termination of pacing, which makes atrial tachycardia very unlikely. The bottom panel shows initiation of the tachycardia with premature atrial contractions (*asterisks*) that makes ventricular tachycardia less likely. The patient went to electrophysiology study and had easily inducible atrioventricular node reentrant tachycardia and underwent slow pathway modification with complete resolution of his episodes of tachycardia. A, atrial; RV, right ventricular; SHOCK, electrogram from the coil; V-A, ventriculoatrial; V-A-V, ventricular-atrial-ventricular.

noise algorithm is called the sensing integrity counter. The sensing integrity counter measures the number of intervals less than 140 ms; if more than 30 episodes are detected within a 3-day window, the criterion is fulfilled. The second noise algorithm is the nonsustained tachycardia log. This criterion is fulfilled if ≥5 sensed events that do not meet detection criteria for therapy are sensed. If any 2 of these 3 criteria are fulfilled, the device is automatically programmed to increase the number of signals required for initial detection of tachycardia to 30/40. Remote monitoring may potentially allow early identification of lead failures. In one analysis of 414 patients with a median follow-up of 3 years, lead failures were identified in 40 (9.7%) patients.[29] The median

time between a diagnostics alert and a lead failure adverse event such as an inappropriate shock was 2.2 days. The investigators calculated that daily remote monitoring would have alerted health care providers of impending lead failure at least 1 day in advance. In another retrospective study of 131 patients with lead fractures, inappropriate shocks occurred in only 21% of patients with the lead integrity alert algorithm compared to 52% of patients whereby this algorithm was not in place.[30] Importantly, remote monitoring decreased the time required to program the ICD off from 15.6 days to 1.5 days when compared with conventional follow-up. Inappropriate shocks were delivered in only 14% of patients with both the lead integrity alert and the remote monitoring.

Table 2
Recall list

Company and Devices (Model Numbers)	Recall Date
Biotronik	
Belos	10/14/2003
Ela/Sorin Alto	7/25/2005
Boston Scientific	
Cognis, Confient, Livian, Prizm, Renewal, Teligen, Vitality	3/19/2010
Guidant (merged with Boston Scientific in 2006)	
Ventak Prizm 2 DR Contak Renewal (H135) and 2 (H155)	7/01/2005
Vitality, Vitality 2 VR, Contak Renewal TR/TR2, Ventak Prizm 2, Insignia, Nexus	07/7/2006
Contak Renewal 3 and 4 (various model numbers) Vitality 2 (various model numbers)	4/5/2007
Contak Renewal 3 AVT CRT-D (multiple models)	3/13/2008
Medtronic	
Micro Jewell II (7223Cx) GEM DR (7271)	4/1/2004
Marquis (7230, 7232, 7274, 7277, 7279) Maximo (7278)	7/7/2005
Sprint Fidelis leads	10/15/2007
St Jude Medical	
Photon (Med V230) Photon Micron (V194, V232) Atlas (V199, V240)	10/06/2005
Epic, Atlas, Convert	1/16/2008
Riata leads Riata ST Silicone leads	12/14/2011
QuickSite LV CRT leads QuickFlex LV CRT leads	4/3/2012

Finally, in a subset of 40 patients in the ECOST study who had Sprint Fidelis leads followed by daily monitoring, lead fracture was identified in 3 patients (7.5%) but only one patient experienced inappropriate shocks.[15]

In December 2011, the FDA issued another large class I recall of defibrillator leads for the St Jude Medical Riata and Riata ST Silicone leads that were initially introduced in 2001. In this case lead failure was due to the conductor wire erosion and externalization through the insulation, termed "inside-out" abrasions. St Jude Medical had stopped selling these leads in late 2010 but unfortunately 227,000 of these leads were implanted worldwide. In an analysis of the Veterans Administration's National Cardiac Device Center Surveillance database, the 5-year failure rate was 2.5%.[31] However, because externalization of conductors is often not associated with changes in electrical parameters, studies that have used fluoroscopy have revealed a higher 15% to 30% rate of abnormal lead appearance consistent with lead insulation breach.[32,33] A recently published retrospective evaluation of 1081 patients with Riata or Riata ST leads found a 6.2% failure rate.[34] Of the lead failures, 70% were associated with abnormal electrical parameters such as increased threshold or noise and 30% were associated with externalized conductors but were electrically intact.[34] In a subset of 110 patients who underwent fluoroscopy, the rate of externalization was 32%, and 30% of leads with externalized conductors had abnormal electrical properties. In April 2012, St Jude voluntarily stopped selling the Quicksite and Quickflex left ventricular leads and the FDA issued a class II recall for these products. In addition, St Jude Medical is performing a comprehensive aftermarket surveillance study on the Durata family of

ICD leads that replaced the Riata family. The Durata family of leads uses the same interior design as the Riata family but is coated with a proprietary Optim insulation that combines silicone and polyurethane. As remote monitoring becomes more accepted and widespread as a method for follow-up, it will become an essential component for surveillance of all leads, but particularly for leads that have been identified with suboptimal performance. However, the impact of remote monitoring will be dependent on the mechanism of lead failure because it depends on development of abnormal measured electrical parameters or the presence of ineffective therapy.

In addition to providing an important component for monitoring a specific patient with a recalled or problematic lead, aggregation of remote monitoring data from large numbers of patients into registries and databanks may be useful for early identification of underperforming leads or generators. In one study, use of a commercially available automatic surveillance system applied retrospectively to a large database of patients with ICD leads was able to identify the higher failure rates associated with the Fidelis lead compared with other ICD leads.[35]

SUMMARY

Over the last decade, remote monitoring has already had an important impact on implantable cardiac device therapy. Randomized clinical trials have consistently found that remote monitoring allows earlier identification of clinical problems and device/hardware problems when compared with traditional in-clinic evaluation. The clinical impact of remote monitoring will depend on the patient and the method of remote monitoring. Remote monitoring will identify more abnormalities in patients with more advanced cardiovascular disease and will be more effective with remote monitoring systems that allow daily measurements, particularly if the measurements are done automatically without patient input. If embraced by physician and patient, and developed correctly, by facilitating communication between patient and provider, remote monitoring will become an integral part of the future of implantable device therapy.

REFERENCES

1. Mond HG, Proclemer A. The 11th world survey of cardiac pacing and implantable cardioverter-defibrillators: calendar year 2009–a World Society of Arrhythmia's project. Pacing Clin Electrophysiol 2011;34:1013–27.

2. Lamas GA, Lee KL, Sweeney MO, et al. Ventricular pacing or dual-chamber pacing for sinus-node dysfunction. N Engl J Med 2002;346:1854–62.

3. Sweeney MO, Ellenbogen KA, Miller EH, et al. The Managed ventricular Pacing™ versus VVI 40 pacing (MVP) trial: clinical background, rationale, design, and implementation. J Cardiovasc Electrophysiol 2006;17:1295–8.

4. Schoenfeld MH, Compton SJ, Mead RH, et al. Remote monitoring of implantable cardioverter defibrillators: a prospective analysis. Pacing Clin Electrophysiol 2004;27:757–63.

5. Crossley GH, Boyle A, Vitense H, et al. The CONNECT (Clinical Evaluation of Remote Notification to Reduce Time to Clinical Decision) trial: the value of wireless remote monitoring with automatic clinician alerts. J Am Coll Cardiol 2011;57:1181–9.

6. Varma N, Epstein AE, Irimpen A, et al. Efficacy and safety of automatic remote monitoring for implantable cardioverter-defibrillator follow-up: the Lumos-T Safely Reduces Routine Office Device Follow-up (TRUST) trial. Circulation 2010;122:325–32.

7. Crossley GH, Chen J, Choucair W, et al. Clinical benefits of remote versus transtelephonic monitoring of implanted pacemakers. J Am Coll Cardiol 2009; 54:2012–9.

8. Cronin EM, Ching EA, Varma N, et al. Remote monitoring of cardiovascular devices: a time and activity analysis. Rhythm 2012;9:1947–51.

9. Varma N, Michalski J, Epstein AE, et al. Automatic remote monitoring of implantable cardioverter-defibrillator lead and generator performance: the Lumos-T Safely RedUceS RouTine Office Device Follow-Up (TRUST) trial. Circ Arrhythm Electrophysiol 2010;3:428–36.

10. Healey JS, Israel CW, Connolly SJ, et al. Relevance of electrical remodeling in human atrial fibrillation: results of the Asymptomatic Atrial Fibrillation and Stroke Evaluation in Pacemaker Patients and the Atrial Fibrillation Reduction Atrial Pacing Trial mechanisms of atrial fibrillation study. Circ Arrhythm Electrophysiol 2012;5:626–31.

11. Sarkar S, Koehler J, Crossley GH, et al. Burden of atrial fibrillation and poor rate control detected by continuous monitoring and the risk for heart failure hospitalization. Am Heart J 2012;164:616–24.

12. Landolina M, Perego GB, Lunati M, et al. Remote monitoring reduces healthcare use and improves quality of care in heart failure patients with implantable defibrillators: the evolution of management strategies of heart failure patients with implantable defibrillators (EVOLVO) study. Circulation 2012;125: 2985–92.

13. Zabel M, Vollmann D, Luthje L, et al. Randomized Clinical evaluatiON of wireless fluid monitoriNg and rEmote ICD managemenT using OptiVol alert-based predefined management to reduce cardiac

decompensation and health care utilization: the CONNECT-OptiVol study. Contemp Clin Trials 2013; 34:109–16.

14. Varma N, Pavri BB, Stambler B, et al. Same-day discovery of implantable cardioverter defibrillator dysfunction in the TRUST remote monitoring trial: influence of contrasting messaging systems. Europace 2013;15(5):697–703.

15. Guedon-Moreau L, Lacroix D, Sadoul N, et al. A randomized study of remote follow-up of implantable cardioverter defibrillators: safety and efficacy report of the ECOST trial. Eur Heart J 2013;34(8): 605–14.

16. Choudhuri I, Desai D, Walburg J, et al. Feasibility of early discharge after implantable cardioverter-defibrillator procedures. J Cardiovasc Electrophysiol 2012;23:1123–9.

17. Preliminary report: effect of encainide and flecainide on mortality in a randomized trial of arrhythmia suppression after myocardial infarction. The Cardiac Arrhythmia Suppression Trial (CAST) Investigators. N Engl J Med 1989;321:406–12.

18. Mason JW. A comparison of electrophysiologic testing with Holter monitoring to predict antiarrhythmic-drug efficacy for ventricular tachyarrhythmias. Electrophysiologic Study versus Electrocardiographic Monitoring Investigators. N Engl J Med 1993;329:445–51.

19. Pacifico A, Hohnloser SH, Williams JH, et al. Prevention of implantable-defibrillator shocks by treatment with sotalol. d, l-Sotalol Implantable Cardioverter-Defibrillator Study Group. N Engl J Med 1999;340: 1855–62.

20. Connolly SJ, Dorian P, Roberts RS, et al. Comparison of beta-blockers, amiodarone plus beta-blockers, or sotalol for prevention of shocks from implantable cardioverter defibrillators: the OPTIC Study: a randomized trial. JAMA 2006;295:165–71.

21. Baquero GA, Banchs JE, Depalma S, et al. Dofetilide reduces the frequency of ventricular arrhythmias and implantable cardioverter defibrillator therapies. J Cardiovasc Electrophysiol 2012;23: 296–301.

22. Dorian P, Al-Khalidi HR, Hohnloser SH, et al. Azimilide reduces emergency department visits and hospitalizations in patients with an implantable cardioverter-defibrillator in a placebo-controlled clinical trial. J Am Coll Cardiol 2008;52:1076–83.

23. Gersak B, Pernat A, Robic B, et al. Low rate of atrial fibrillation recurrence verified by implantable loop recorder monitoring following a convergent epicardial and endocardial ablation of atrial fibrillation. J Cardiovasc Electrophysiol 2012;23: 1059–66.

24. Pokushalov E, Romanov A, Cherniavsky A, et al. Ablation of paroxysmal atrial fibrillation during coronary artery bypass grafting: 12 months' follow-up

through implantable loop recorder. Eur J Cardiothorac Surg 2011;40:405–11.

25. Hayes DL, Graham KJ, Irwin M, et al. A multicenter experience with a bipolar tined polyurethane ventricular lead. Pacing Clin Electrophysiol 1992;15: 1033–9.

26. Ellenbogen KA, Wood MA, Shepard RK, et al. Detection and management of an implantable cardioverter defibrillator lead failure: incidence and clinical implications. J Am Coll Cardiol 2003;41: 73–80.

27. Urgent medical device information. Sprint Fidelis lead patient management. Minneapolis (MN): Medtronic; 2007 [Physician letter].

28. Hauser RG, Hayes DL. Increasing hazard of Sprint Fidelis implantable cardioverter-defibrillator lead failure. Heart Rhythm 2009;6:605–10.

29. Ricci RP, Pignalberi C, Magris B, et al. Can we predict and prevent adverse events related to high-voltage implantable cardioverter defibrillator lead failure? J Interv Card Electrophysiol 2012;33:113–21.

30. Blanck Z, Axtell K, Brodhagen K, et al. Inappropriate shocks in patients with Fidelis(R) lead fractures: impact of remote monitoring and the lead integrity algorithm. J Cardiovasc Electrophysiol 2011;22: 1107–14.

31. Sung RK, Massie BM, Varosy PD, et al. Long-term electrical survival analysis of Riata and Riata ST silicone leads: National Veterans Affairs experience. Heart Rhythm 2012;9(12):1954–61.

32. Kodoth VN, Hodkinson EC, Noad RL, et al. Fluoroscopic and electrical assessment of a series of defibrillation leads: prevalence of externalized conductors. Pacing Clin Electrophysiol 2012;35:1498–504.

33. Theuns DA, Elvan A, de Voogt W, et al. Prevalence and presentation of externalized conductors and electrical abnormalities in riata defibrillator leads after fluoroscopic screening: report from the Netherlands heart rhythm association device advisory committee. Circ Arrhythm Electrophysiol 2012;5:1059–63.

34. Abdelhadi RH, Saba SF, Ellis CR, et al. Independent multicenter study of Riata and Riata ST implantable cardioverter-defibrillator leads. Heart Rhythm 2013; 10(3):361–5.

35. Hauser RG, Mugglin AS, Friedman PA, et al. Early detection of an underperforming implantable cardiovascular device using an automated safety surveillance tool. Circ Cardiovasc Qual Outcomes 2012; 5:189–96.

36. Mabo P, Victor F, Bazin P, et al. A randomized trial of long-term remote monitoring of pacemaker recipients (the COMPAS trial). Eur Heart J 2012;33: 1105–11.

37. Mabo P. EVATEL: remote follow-up of patients implanted with an ICD. Paris: European Society of Cardiology (ESC) Congress; 2011.

Physiologic Sensors in Pacemakers
How Do They Work and How Many Do We Need?

Will W. Xiong, MD, PhD, David G. Benditt, MD*

KEYWORDS

- Physical sensor • Rate adaptation • Pacemaker • Hemodynamic sensor

KEY POINTS

- Sensor-based rate adaptation is an essential part of modern cardiac pacing therapy.
- The benefits of rate-adaptive ventricular pacing in comparison with fixed-rate ventricular pacing have been demonstrated in many clinical studies, but the additional benefit of rate adaptation in dual-chamber pacemaker systems (DDDR vs DDD) has not been clearly established despite large clinical studies.
- The advantage of dual-sensor or multiple-sensor systems over a single sensor is not yet certain and likely varies depending on specific patient cohorts.
- The advantage of dual-/multiple-sensor pacing is more likely to be obtained in patients with an active lifestyle. Whether the complexity of such systems (ie, requiring more attention to programming and their added cost) outweigh any physiologic benefit are questions that are not likely to be resolved for some time.
- The future direction of hemodynamic sensors will be toward reliable assessment of crucial hemodynamic variables such as preload, afterload, left ventricular ejection fraction and stroke volume.

INTRODUCTION

The first implantable cardiac pacemakers were designed to pace at a fixed rate without sensing the patient's intrinsic heart rhythm. These fixed-rate devices were primarily used for ventricular pacing (VVI mode); atrial pacing (AAI mode) was a possibility if atrioventricular conduction was adequate, but was only rarely attempted by most implanters owing to instability of passive-fixation endocardial pacing leads, and both the difficulty in implantation and poor longevity of epicardial pacing leads (**Box 1**). Subsequently, devices that sensed native atrial activity were introduced (eg, VDI, DDD modes) in conjunction with active-fixation lead technologies. These latter pulse-generator and lead systems provided a more physiologic approach to pacing, but their rate-adaptive capability was undermined by the frequent presence of native and/or drug-induced sinus node dysfunction in many paced patients. Furthermore, in the presence of permanent atrial fibrillation or other atrial tachycardias, atrial electrical activity was not a desirable sensing option.

W.W.X. is supported by a Fellowship grant from the Cardiac Arrhythmia Center, Cardiovascular Division, University of Minnesota.
Conflicts of Interest: W.W.X., None; D.G.B., Consultant and equity: Medtronic Inc, St Jude Medical Inc.
Cardiovascular Division, Cardiac Arrhythmia Center, University of Minnesota School of Medicine, Mail Code 508, 420 Delaware Street Southeast, Minneapolis, MN 55436, USA
* Corresponding author.
E-mail address: bendi001@umn.edu

Card Electrophysiol Clin 5 (2013) 303–316
http://dx.doi.org/10.1016/j.ccep.2013.05.007
1877-9182/13/$ – see front matter © 2013 Elsevier Inc. All rights reserved.

cardiacEP.theclinics.com

Box 1
Pacing modes cited in this article
AAI	Atrial pacing; atrial sensing and inhibition
AAIR	Atrial pacing; atrial sensing and inhibition; rate-modulated pacing
VVI	Ventricular pacing; ventricular sensing and inhibition
VVIR	Ventricular pacing; ventricular sensing and inhibition; rate-modulated pacing
DDD	Dual-chamber pacing; dual-chamber sensing and inhibition; tracking of the atrium
DDDR	Dual-chamber pacing; dual-chamber sensing and inhibition; tracking of the atrium; atrioventricular sequential rate modulation
DVI	Dual-chamber pacing; ventricular sensing and inhibition; no tracking of the atrium
DVIR	Dual-chamber pacing; ventricular sensing and inhibition; no tracking of the atrium; atrioventricular sequential rate modulation

The first sensor-based rate-adaptive pacemaker was introduced in the 1970s by Italian researchers, and used alterations of blood pH during exercise to effect changes in pacing rate.[1] This system did not become widely used, but the concept triggered subsequent technological development, and rate-adaptive pacing systems using one or other form of "physiologic" sensor began to receive broad acceptance in clinical practice in the mid-1980s. Not only have a wide variety of sensor systems been developed, but sensor combinations have also been introduced in an attempt to optimize physiologic benefits.[2,3] This article reviews the technology and clinical utility of the most widely used rate-adaptive sensor systems and sensor system combinations for implantable cardiac pacemakers.

SENSORS FOR RATE-ADAPTIVE PACING

In the 1980s[4] physiologic sensors were categorized into 5 groups based on the accuracy of their relationship to oxygen consumption: (1) those measuring oxygen consumption directly, such as oxygen uptake; (2) sensors having a linear relationship with the sensors of the first group, such as cardiac output, atrioventricular oxygen difference, or minute ventilation (MV)[5,6]; (3) those having a linear relationship with sensors of the second group, such as heart rate, stroke volume,

mixed oxygen saturation, tidal volume, or respiratory rate[7,8]; (4) sensors dependent on sympathetic activity and circulation catecholamines, such as right ventricular dP/dt and QT interval[9]; and (5) those using physiologic feedback from metabolism, such as mixed venous lactate and bicarbonate levels or central venous pH.[10] Subsequent work introduced an additional group of physical sensors that corresponded at best only indirectly to metabolic state, but rather more directly on body movement (ie, activity sensors and accelerometers).[11–13]

Despite the great variety of sensors that have been designed and investigated in the past, only a few sensors for rate-adaptive application proved to be commercially successful and remain clinically available. Activity sensing (mainly accelerometer-based), MV (respiration-based), and so-called closed-loop stimulation sensors using electrical bioimpedance are currently the primary surviving systems. Sensors for QT interval (more accurately termed Stim-T interval) detection or peak endocardial acceleration (PEA) are much less widely used.

Activity Sensors

Sensors capable of responding in a more or less graduated fashion to vibration or acceleration forces applied to the pacemaker body by surrounding tissues are referred to as activity sensors. Activity sensing is most frequently used for rate-adaptive pacing, in large part because of its simplicity in application, robustness, and compatibility with standard pacing leads. Although these may be the least "physiologic" sensors, they exhibit high reliability as well as excellent long-term stability.

The first activity sensor used in a commercially successful pacemaker (Activitrax; Medtronic Inc, Minneapolis, MN, USA; **Fig. 1**A) was a piezoelectric crystal designed to detect vibration generated by body movement.[14] The vibration of the human body, and in particular the muscle mass and skeleton in proximity to the pacemaker, are detected by a piezoelectric crystal bonded to the interior surface of the pulse generator casing that faces the pectoral muscle (see **Fig. 1**B). Vibration is sensed from mechanical forces through tissue/skeleton contact. The slight deformation of the piezoelectric crystal generates a small electric voltage. Depending on a predetermined programmable threshold and the extent of body motion, the voltage may be large enough to be counted as signals and be used for triggering alterations in the pacing rate. The amount of tissue contact and the coupling mass of mechanical force in each

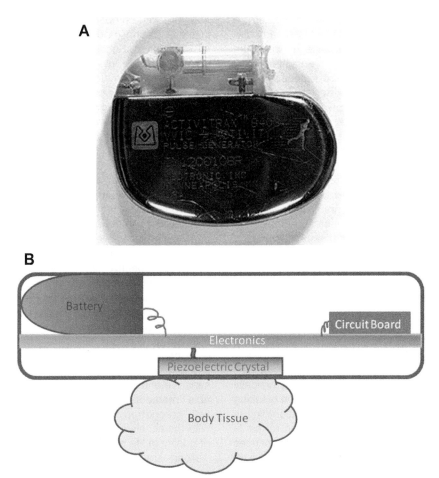

Fig. 1. (*A*) The first commercially successful activity-sensor–based pacemaker. (*B*) Vibration-triggered activity sensor using the piezoelectric crystal. The piezoelectric crystal is bound to the interior surface of the activity sensor, and can sense the tissue vibration via mechanical forces transmitted from the surrounding tissue. (Photo in Panel [*A*], *Courtesy of* Medtronic Inc, Minneapolis, MN.)

individual may vary substantially and, consequently, techniques have been proposed to individualize sensor programming.[12]

Body movement can also be detected by an accelerometer (typically a piezoelectric element, but other technologies could be used), which for this application is usually mounted on the hybrid circuitry of the pulse generator and structurally shielded from the pulse-generator casing (**Fig. 2**). Thus, in contrast to the vibration-detector piezoelectric crystal, the accelerometer is independent of mechanical forces from tissue contact. However, it is still influenced by body movement. The motion perpendicular to the plane of an accelerometer yields the electrical signal for changes in the heart rate.

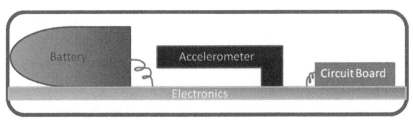

Fig. 2. Activity sensor using an accelerometer. The accelerometer is mounted on a hybrid circuitry and structurally removed from the pacemaker casing. The sensor is thereby unaffected by mechanical forces transmitted from the surrounding tissue, but is subject to forces generated by physical body movement.

Apart from the manner in which the accelerometer is mounted within the device (as already discussed), the other main difference between the piezoelectric crystal vibration system and accelerometer is how the signals are processed. The vibration-based system was designed to count only those signals above a given programmable voltage threshold for purposes of assessing "activity level," whereas the accelerometer-based systems evolved to integrate the voltage of signals from the sensor element, with the expectation that this would allow a more proportional rate response to exercise. For example, contrary to the predetermined but programmable activity-sensing thresholds in the vibration-application piezoelectric crystal, a rolling threshold is used in an accelerometer of current Medtronic devices. The rolling threshold is a function of both the frequency of counts surpassing the detection threshold and the amplitude of these counts. Therefore, an accelerometer tends to reduce the detection of low-intensity but high-frequency accelerations during riding in a motor vehicle, but permits detection of high-intensity signals during physical exercise. Body motion with recurring patterns such as bicycle riding or walking typically falls in the range of 1 to 4 Hz.[11] Vibration resulting from nonexertion such as motor vehicle riding is usually more than 10 Hz. The limitation to the 1- to 10-Hz range in the accelerometer enhances the specificity of responses to signals derived from physical activities.

Walking upstairs or downstairs tends to result in acceleration frequency of less than 4 Hz. Sophisticated signal processing can further differentiate these 2 different activities. With 72 to 120 steps/min, walking upstairs or downstairs yields a heart rate of 117 to 132 beats/min or 82 to 109 beats/min, respectively.[15] On the other hand, physicians can predetermine Activity of Daily Living (ADL) rates for patients based on previously stored data to offer reasonable heart-rate increments for modest physical activity associated with daily chores.

Cardiac pacing with activity-sensor systems for rate adaptation has been shown to provide an improvement in exercise capacity and reduction in symptoms in clinical investigations. Benditt and colleagues[3] demonstrated physiologic benefits of a single-chamber ventricular pacing system using a piezoceramic sensor for rate adaptation. Compared with findings during fixed-rate VVI pacing, VVIR pacing was associated with greater exercise-induced positive chronotropic response, prolongation of exercise duration, increased peak oxygen consumption, and onset of anaerobic threshold at a higher oxygen consumption.[3] In addition, with comparable exercise stages tested in the 2 pacing modes, perceived exertion was lower during VVIR than with VVI pacing. Of interest, other crossover investigations comparing VVIR and DDD pacing modes yield no significant difference in symptom scores, maximal exercise performance, or oxygen consumption.[16,17]

The roles of the vibratory activity sensor, the accelerometer application, or a blended sensor (ie, with the addition of a second sensor technology) in rate-adaptive pacing are evolving. However, there is increased preference for the accelerometer over the vibration approach. Compared with the vibration sensor, the accelerometer-based pacemakers were found to provide better sinus rate approximation as well as better rate adaptation during treadmill exercises.[18,19] In a subsequent larger retrospective study, the quality of life did not differ between patients with the vibration system and those with an accelerometer as an activity sensor, although it appeared to be worse in the patients with blended sensors.[20]

In the randomized LIFE trial, a blended sensor (a response factor of 8 for the accelerometer and a response factor of 4 for the MV sensor; 1 = least sensitive and 16 = most sensitive) showed favorable metabolic-chronotropic slope in patients with chronotropic incompetence in comparison with the accelerometer alone, although measures of quality of life remained unchanged.[21]

Apart from their rate-adaptive use, activity sensors offer additional advantages in implanted devices. These sensors are used to obtain a general sense of patients' levels of physical activity. Such assessments have proved helpful in both pacemakers and implantable cardiac defibrillators (ICDs) for evaluation of the impact of altering disease state (particularly heart failure) on quality of life. For instance, reduction of activity in conjunction with decreased transpulmonary bioimpedance (eg, OptiVol; Medtronic Inc) (**Fig. 3**)[22] or increased daily weight (Latitude; Boston Scientific, St Paul, MN, USA) would tend to signal worsening heart-failure status and need for adjustment of medical therapy.

Although clinically widely used and commercially available from several manufacturers, the activity-sensor concept has important limitations. For example, direct pressure on a piezoelectric crystal (such as may occur if a patient lies in a prone position pressing on the device) may cause a false-positive rate response, particularly with a vibration-based device. In fact, positive feedback may occur as the device senses vibrations generated by the patient's own heart and interprets it to be external physical activity; a resulting increased pacing rate may lead to a further upward ramp in

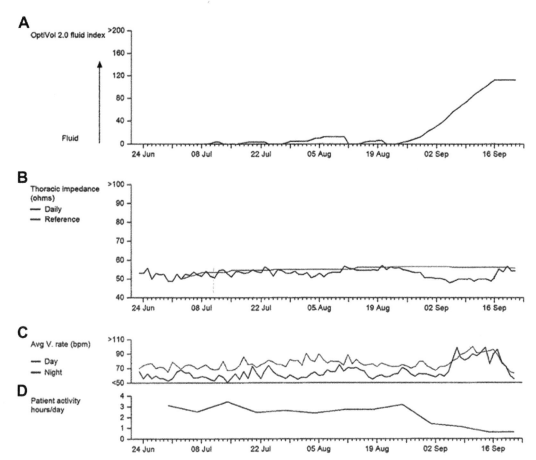

Fig. 3. Comparison of OptiVol fluid index, thoracic impedance, night heart rate, and daily activity before admission for congestive heart failure in a patient with a Medtronic ICD. (*A*) OptiVol fluid index started to escalate approximately 3 weeks before admission (*dashed line*). OptiVol 2.0 fluid index is an accumulation of the difference between the daily and reference impedance. (*B*) Thoracic impedance concurrently decreased. (*C*) The night heart rate increased before hospital admission. (*D*) Daily activity was reduced simultaneously as the OptiVol fluid index rose.

rate until the programmed maximum allowable sensor rate is achieved. An additional disadvantage of activity sensing is its low proportionality to the level of workload.[23] Body motion does not necessarily translate into work intensity. Climbing stairs leads to a lower acceleration signal compared with descending the stairs.[24,25] Similarly, activity that generates a less jarring effect on the body (eg, swimming, or running on a soft surface) may not elicit a sufficient heart-rate response in comparison with activities that cause more skeletal vibration (eg, running on a hard surface). Finally, activity sensing may not detect isometric exercise optimally, and would not be expected to react appropriately in terms of heart-rate change in response to emotional stress.[26]

Minute Ventilation Sensor

MV is a reliable physiologic indicator that has been demonstrated to have an excellent correlation

with metabolic demand[4,27]; this measure is the product of respiratory rate and tidal volume. Comparative studies of the MV and the activity-sensor pacing systems in the same patients have demonstrated that the MV system more closely parallels normal sinus response to activity.[6] MV has been shown to almost correlate linearly with heart rate.[28,29]

The modern respiratory sensor detects electrical bioimpedance as a surrogate measure of MV. Impedance is a measure of factors opposing the flow of electric current and is derived from resistivity to an injected subthreshold electric current across the tissue. The measurement is typically accomplished by injecting a very small and short-duration current from the pacemaker can to the pacing lead, where a resulting voltage is measured. An estimate of the transthoracic impedance is then calculated, based on the known current and the measured voltage. For this application, conventional respiratory sensor systems only require a standard bipolar lead in the right atrium or ventricle, without other specialized hardware.

The MV sensor's output is approximately proportional to oxygen consumption below anaerobic threshold. In this regard, it is significantly better in accomplishing a near-normal pacing rate–workload relationship in comparison with the activity sensor.[5] Clinical study has also demonstrated that when compared with VVI pacing, MV-based VVIR pacing improved exercise capacity by 33% (from 437 ± 42 seconds in the VVI mode to 593 ± 57 seconds in VVIR mode), symptomatology, and maximal oxygen consumption.[5]

The MV sensor has limitations. Compared with an activity sensor, the initial onset of rate adaptation at the beginning of exercise is slower with the MV sensor. False-positive reactions may occur in response to electromagnetic interference, arm swinging, hyperventilation (related for instance to anxiety or respiratory diseases), or even coughing.

Closed-Loop Stimulation Sensor

A rate-adaptation circuit requires an algorithm that modulates the pacing rate in response to changes in physical or physiologic changes detected by the sensor(s) being used. However, often because of the variable magnitude of rate adaptation that

occurs among individuals, the algorithm needs adjustment either manually by programming or by some form of automatic optimization of the rate-adaptation settings. In the best circumstance, changes in the measured sensor output diminish as the heart rate is adjusted toward optimal physiologic value for the specific metabolic circumstances of the moment. This form of negative feedback is characteristic of properly operating closed-loop control systems. However, in the pacing realm, not all sensor systems are capable of such operation.

In open-loop stimulation, there is an absence of feedback induced by changes monitored by sensors. Such is the case with activity sensors whereby activity-induced increased pacing rate does not intrinsically result in a reduction of the physiologic driving signal (ie, increased heart rate does not diminish the vibrations). Conversely, in the closed-loop sensor system, the alterations in parameters identified by the sensor (ie, the surrogate of myocardial contractile drive) leads to a negative feedback of the rate-adaptation response (ie, because increased rate reduces need for elevated myocardial contractile activity) with minimal programming (**Fig. 4**).

The currently commercially available closed-loop stimulation sensor system (Biotronik Inc,

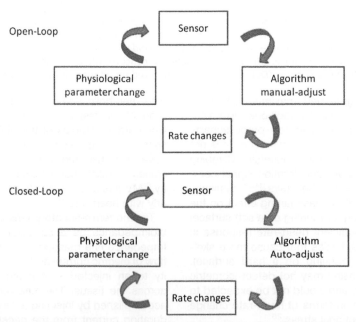

Fig. 4. Open-loop and closed-loop sensors. In open-loop sensor systems, the physiologic changes detected by the sensor are translated to the changes in the rate via an algorithm. Optimization of the sensor requires the physician's input. The rate changes do not have a negative feedback to the physiologic parameters. In closed-loop sensor systems, the physiologic changes identified by the sensor are converted to the rate changes, the latter of which leads to changes in the physiologic parameter in the opposite direction. Thus these systems exhibit a negative feedback of alteration of heart rate on the sensed variable.

Berlin, Germany) measures the electrical bioimpedance from the tip of a right ventricular unipoloar lead to the pacemaker can (see earlier discussion). For the most part, the measured impedance reflects the near-field effects of change in right ventricular volumes, thereby roughly reflecting myocardial "contractile" state.

Based on the electrode location and the theory that proximate tissues or blood contribute more to bioimpedance than do remote tissues, the measured alterations of the unipolar right ventricular impedance during the cardiac cycle correlates with the varied content of blood (low impedance) and tissue (high impedance) around the tip of the pacing electrode. During myocardial contraction, the impedance continuously rises, reaching its maximum in late systole. This impedance increase correlates with right ventricular contractile state, thereby serving as a surrogate of the inotropic state of the heart.[30] During exercise cardiac contractility is enhanced excessively in the absence of an appropriately increased heart rate, to cope with increased metabolic demand. If, however, the pacing system is able to provide sufficient rate response, the necessary contractile increase is diminished much as it would be had the native normal chronotropic response been present, thereby providing a negative feedback loop owing to the nature of the sensed variable.

In the case of the bioimpedance closed-loop system, myocardial contractile state or its bioimpedance surrogate is by itself the presumed sensed variable. Although this may not be precisely the case from a physiologic perspective, it seems close enough for operational purposes. A limitation would be disease states that affect the ventricular apex and/or septum such as prior myocardial infarctions or cardiomyopathy. On the other hand, it should be very effective in healthy hearts. This method has therefore been proposed to be useful for triggering pacing in patients with vasovagal syncope (most often younger patients with healthy hearts), a condition whereby increased myocardial contractile state is believed to be a physiologic trigger.[31] However, further evidence is needed before this application can be considered as valid for such patients.

Peak Endocardial Acceleration

An approximation of cardiac contractility can be obtained by measuring the maximal velocity of shortening of the adjacent myocardium with a catheter-tip accelerometer in the ventricle. To this end, a microaccelerometer placed at the tip of a ventricular pacing lead is used to detect PEA. The microaccelerometer quantifies the amplitude of myocardial vibration during the isovolumetric contraction phase of the cardiac cycle. The lead is placed against the right ventricular wall so that, at least theoretically, the accelerometer is relatively insensitive to ventricular pressure but very sensitive to myocardial acceleration.

PEA has been shown to exhibit good correlation with estimates of myocardial contractile state during cardiac isometric systolic contraction (dP/dt_{max}). These correlations have been shown with increased sympathetic activity resulting from both physical and mental stress, and with physiologic heart-rate modulation during daily life activities including exercise.[32,33]

As was the case with the closed-loop electrical bioimpedance sensor discussed earlier, PEA could in theory also be used in a closed-loop fashion for the management of patients with vasovagal syncope.[34] The increase in sympathetic activity before vasovagal syncope may be sensed by a lead-tip microaccelerometer in the right ventricle, and used to drive a rate-adaptive pacer. Furthermore, a device equipped with an implantable sensor capable of measuring PEA has also been used to monitor cardiac function and guide cardiac resynchronization therapy (CRT) programming.[35] A new CRT optimization algorithm was developed, based on recording of PEA, which reflects greatest left ventricular dP/dt_{max}, to identify an optimized CRT configuration.

Miscellaneous Sensors

Several sensor systems other than those discussed to this point have been introduced into implantable devices over the years.[10,33,36] Despite often superior physiologic potential, most of these innovations failed to achieve commercial acceptance and thus vanished. In each case, the most important liability was the need for a special pacing lead on which the sensor was placed. Inasmuch as conventional pacing leads remain the Achilles heel of implantable pacemakers, the need for even more complex leads is a major liability.

A venous temperature-based system was approved for use in the United States (Kelvin; Cook Pacemakers Corp, Leechburg, PA). The lead contained a temperature detector, and the rate was adjusted based on an algorithm that was moderately complex and required specific adjustment, particularly in the initial phase of exercise.

An oxygen-sensing system initially received considerable interest, based on clinical evaluation in Scandinavia, but was ultimately abandoned for rate-adaptive applications. Again, the placement of the oxygen sensor on the lead created considerable concern regarding long-term integrity of the pacing lead. Other issues regarding sensor stability, such as the sensor being covered by fibrous tissue over time, have also raised concern.

A right ventricular pressure-sensing system suffered a similar fate. In this case not only was the lead complex in terms of construction, but the possibility that the sensor would change its characteristic performance over time, given the possibility of overgrowth by tissue, was an additional worry.

Combination of Sensors

Why may a single sensor not be enough?

As already noted, each individual sensor technology has its advantages but also comes with often crucial disadvantages. Mimicking normal sinus node behavior by pacemaker rate adaptation involves a complex process beyond the capability of any single sensor. The activity sensors using piezoelectric crystals with an algorithm that relies on peak counting (ie, the number of activity signals generated that surpass in amplitude/strength the physician-preprogrammed threshold) do not typically discriminate well among varied levels of exercise. Thus, an activity sensor alone, while very responsive at onset of exertion, is not reliably proportional to cardiac workload during sustained exercise. Furthermore, an activity sensor is ineffective in assessing emotional changes and is relatively poor in assessing isometric exercise. On the other hand, although the MV sensor exhibits relatively good correlation with workload,[5] it has relatively slow responsiveness at exercise onset.[37,38] Consequently, the rapid-response sensor is not proportional, but a proportional sensor does not respond sufficiently quickly. Therefore, the combination of 2 (or more) sensors is conceptually a reasonable choice, and several combined sensor-based devices currently exist.

There are, in general terms, 2 modalities whereby a combination of sensors operates. First, sensor cross-checking refers to nullifying or diminishing the response of rate adaptation by a more sensitive yet less specific sensor in the absence of registration of physical or emotional stress by a more specific sensor. Sensor cross-checking prevents false-positive rate acceleration. Second, sensor blending represents either a combination of sensors in a certain ratio or "faster wins," the latter of which denotes that the higher rate of either sensor is the rate that is chosen. As such, a rapidly reacting sensor (eg, activity sensor) is used at the onset of exercise, and the slow-reacting sensor (eg, MV sensor) adjusts the heart-rate proportionally during prolonged workload and is ultimately expected to take over as exercise persists.

Combined activity and QT (Stim-T)

The algorithms for sensor combinations of activity with QT sensors have both sensor cross-checking (**Fig. 5**) and sensor blending. In sensor blending, activity and QT are programmed with various ratios. The blending results in a rapid response at the onset of exercise and proportional rate adaptation during sustained exertion (**Fig. 6**).

The initial stage of exercise is dominated by the activity sensing, and the subsequent stage of exercise is mainly modulated by the QT input. The activity sensor alone tends to "overpace" compared with QT sensors.[39] The combined sensing capability, however, produces a more gradual increase in pacing rate.[40] Because the QT sensor has higher specificity for physiologic changes, it offers very reliable sensor cross-checking. Sensor cross-checking has been demonstrated to prevent a sustained high pacing rate caused by false-positive activity sensing (tapping, vibrating pacemaker, or static pressure).[40] Dual-sensor pacing has been shown to achieve a better heart rate to workload relationship compared with single-sensor operation, and yields a cardiac response without overpacing or using contractility reserve during exercise.[41]

Combined activity and minute ventilation

Commercially, this sensor combination has proved to be the most successful. The integration of activity and MV sensors gives rise to a quick initial response and enhances the proportionality of rate response to higher workload. Activity sensors and MV sensors can cross-check each other.

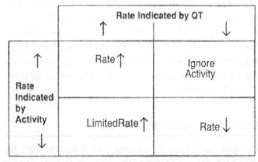

Fig. 5. Sensor cross-checking. Effective changes in the pacing rate produced by a combination of QT and activity sensoring. (*From* Connelly DT. Initial experience with a new single chamber, dual sensor rate responsive pacemaker. The Topaz Study Group. Pacing Clin Electrophysiol 1993;16:1834; with permission.)

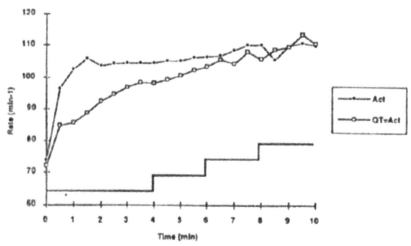

Fig. 6. Rate response during chronotropic assessment exercise protocol in 15 patients, comparing response in dual-sensor mode and activity-only mode. (*From* Connelly DT. Initial experience with a new single chamber, dual sensor rate responsive pacemaker. The Topaz Study Group. Pacing Clin Electrophysiol 1993;16:1837; with permission.)

In the absence of the MV sensor indicating exercise, activity sensor-driven pacing is limited to only achieving a moderate rate increase to daily activity of living (ADL) rates, rather than the maximal rate. The converse also holds true. It has been shown that the integrated sensor mode with an automatic rate profile optimization algorithm led to a faster speed of rate response with a shorter delay time.[42] Furthermore, the maximal sensor rates were significantly more proportional to workload for the combined sensor systems when compared with either the activity or MV sensing alone. Thus, the combination of activity and MV can improve rate-response profiles during exercise and ADLs un comparison with the individual sensor response.[42] In patients with chronotropic incompetence, a blended sensor has been shown to exhibit a favorable metabolic chronotropic relationship when compared with an accelerometer alone, although the quality of life remains unchanged.[21]

How many sensors are needed for rate-response pacing?

At present, the combined-activity and MV sensors are the most commonly used dual sensors for rate adaptation (eg, Medtronic Kappa 400 and Boston Scientific Insignia). Closed-loop stimulation in combination with an activity sensor is also clinically available (eg, Evia; Biotronik). Cross-checking is very frequently used, whereas blending is used less often depending on the various models.

A clinical benefit of a dual sensor over a single sensor has been shown in several small studies[42,43]; however, evidence from large-scale randomized investigation is lacking. Nevertheless, in patients with a very active lifestyle, the dual sensors for rate-response pacing are likely to offer clinical benefit.

Clinical Outcomes of Rate-Response Pacing

Compared with fixed-rate pacing, rate-adaptive single-chamber ventricular (VVIR) pacing has shown advantages in both heart rate and exercise capacity. Better quality of life has been observed in VVIR pacing compared with VVI mode.[43] However, patients with atrial-based rate-adaptive pacing (AAIR) mode had an even better quality of life than VVIR patients in an early study.[44] On the other hand, persistent concerns remain regarding AAIR mode[45]; these include progressive atrioventricular conduction diseases, lack of atrioventricular adaptation (ie, excessive PR-interval prolongation at high pacing rates), and potential Wenckebach atrioventricular block induced by high atrial pacing rates.

With regard to comparison of DDDR benefits over DDD mode, the crucial factors are high right ventricular pacing burden and potential impact on ventricular function over the long term (about 25% of ventricular-paced patients exhibit left ventricular dysfunction over time, but who is susceptible cannot be predicted). In the short term, differences, if any, appear to be minor. For instance, in a study involving 873 patients, there were no differences in exercise capacity despite an increase in the average heart rate from 101 beats/min to 113 beats/min over a period of 6 months.[46] Ventricular pacing of more than 90% was registered in both modes.

Minimizing ventricular pacing might be helpful in reducing the impact of a high sensor-driven pacing burden. Moreover, a different right ventricular pacing site other than right ventricular apex may be helpful; studies with pacing at the right ventricular septum have shown improved left ventricular ejection fraction and exercise capacity[47] in comparison with the right ventricular apex. Right ventricular septal pacing improved left systolic and diastolic function and 6-minute walk at 18 months in patients with previously permanent right ventricular apical pacing, suggesting potential reversal of the detrimental effects of right ventricular apical pacing.

HEMODYNAMIC SENSORS FOR CARDIAC PACING IN PATIENTS WITH HEART FAILURE

Diagnostic markers that may be useful for monitoring patients with heart failure can be derived from pacemaker electrograms; such markers include heart rate variability, percentage of biventricular pacing, atrial fibrillation duration/burden, presence and severity of ventricular arrhythmia, night heart rate, and daily activity monitoring.[22] Other methods include measurement of right ventricular pressure, left atrial pressure, and pulmonary arterial pressure.

Peak Endocardial Acceleration

As mentioned earlier, PEA can assess endocardial motion/tension detected by a microaccelerometer placed at the tip of a ventricular pacing lead. The PEA correlates well with myocardial contractility during the cardiac isometric systolic contraction (dP/dt_{max}), and is a capable surrogate reflecting sympathetic activity with both physical and mental stress.[32,33]

The amplitude of PEA also parallels left ventricular maximal dP/dt. The first PEA was recorded 150 milliseconds after the R wave, representing the isovolumic contraction phase of the left ventricle (PEA-I). A small signal, designated as PEA-II, occurs during isovolumic relaxation and is recorded in the 100-millisecond period after the T wave (**Fig. 7**).[48] The magnitude of PEA-II is associated with velocity of changes in the pressure gradient across the aortic valve at the time of valve closure. Thus, PEA-II reflects the rate of ventricular pressure drop (negative dP/dt) and aortic diastolic pressure. It is interesting that the peak-to-peak myocardial vibration known as PEA signals was found to be also measured reliably in the right atrium.[49] The amplitude of PEA in the right atrium was smaller but proportional to that in the right ventricle, suggesting that PEA possibly

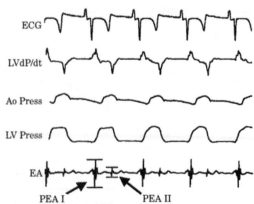

Fig. 7. Typical electrocardiograph (ECG), left ventricular dP/dt (LVdP/dt), aortic pressure (Ao Press), left ventricular pressure (LV Press), and accelerometer (EA) tracings. The peak of the accelerometer tracing (PEA-I) occurs during the isovolumic systole in a 150-millisecond interval following the R wave on ECG. The peak of the accelerometer tracing during the isovolumic diastole (PEA-II) occurs in a 100-millisecond period following the T wave on ECG. (*From* Plicchi G, Marcelli E, Parlapiano M, et al. PEA I and PEA II based implantable haemodynamic monitor: preclinical studies in sheep. Europace 2002;4:51; with permission.)

reflected global ventricular contractility independent of the recording site.[49]

Intrathoracic Impedance

Intrathoracic impedance is estimated by injecting a small current from the pacemaker body to the defibrillator lead in the right ventricular apex (**Fig. 8**). Among the various impedance-current vectors that could be chosen, the right ventricular coil to the device case appears to be the best. In one report, intrathoracic impedance started to

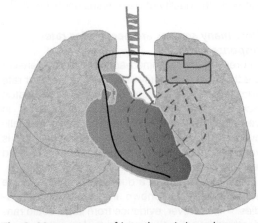

Fig. 8. Measurement of intrathoracic impedance.

decline 15.3 ± 10.6 days before the onset of worsening symptoms of heart failure (pulmonary congestion). By contrast, the earliest clinical warning provided by worsening dyspnea became evident only about 3 days before admission.[50] There was an inverse correlation between intrathoracic impedance and pulmonary capillary wedge pressure, as well as between intrathoracic impedance and net fluid loss with diuretics during hospitalization. Detection of impedance reduction was 76.9% sensitive (threshold crossing at 60 Ω/d) in detecting hospitalization for fluid overload, with 1.5 false-positive detections per patient-year of follow-up.

The effectiveness of Automatic OptiVol alert (Medtronic) was investigated in the Italian OptiVol study.[51] Sixty-seven percent of patients with heart failure were detected when OptiVol alert was enabled. By contrast, hospitalization for heart failure was significantly increased (20% vs 7%) when the OptiVol alert was disabled, suggesting that the alert capability could be useful to decrease the number of heart-failure hospitalizations by allowing timely detection and outpatient therapeutic intervention. Furthermore, intrathoracic impedance may be a better clinical marker than daily weight monitoring in patients with heart failure. In one report, OptiVol crossing had a higher sensitivity (76% vs 23%) for detection of heart failure in comparison with weight monitoring.[52]

Intracardiac Ventricular Impedance

In contrast to intrathoracic impedance that attempts to measure pulmonary fluid status, intracardiac ventricular impedance can provide estimates of left ventricular volume by the addition of a left ventricular lead in CRT systems. Unlike intrathoracic impedance, which needs approximately 1 month for device pocket maturation because of local tissue edema, there is minimal time delay with intraventricular impedance. Intrathoracic impedance is adversely affected by pleural effusion and pneumonia, whereas intracardiac ventricular impedance is much less disturbed.

Unipolar impedance has been recorded from the closed-loop stimulation sensor in the right ventricular apex. The signals only represent a regional contractility rather than stroke volume.[53] Multipolar impedance with incorporation of a left ventricular vector significantly improves assessment of changes in left ventricular volume in heart failure.

Biventricular impedance has been studied in a rapid pacing-induced experimental model of heart failure.[54] Stroke impedance was defined as the difference between systolic and diastolic impedance.

Systolic impedance reflects the highest impedance 50 to 500 milliseconds after the R wave. Diastolic impedance is measured by a 20-millisecond window within the R wave. The increase in left ventricular diastolic pressure was found to correlate well with the diastolic impedance, but has a poorer correlation with intrathoracic impedance. Clinical study has demonstrated a good correlation between stroke impedance and stroke volume or pulse pressure.[55]

SUMMARY

Sensor-based rate adaptation is an essential part of modern cardiac pacing therapy. The benefits of rate-adaptive ventricular in comparison with fixed-rate ventricular pacing have been demonstrated in many clinical studies. On the other hand, the additional benefit of rate adaptation in dual-chamber pacemaker systems (DDDR vs DDD) has not been clearly established despite large clinical studies. The absence of evident advantage might be related to excessive sensor-driven right ventricular pacing, or the subtle differences between absent and nearly normal sensor-based chronotropic response in most day-to-day activities. Whether alternative pacing sites in the right ventricle would affect outcomes remains to be determined.

Finally, the advantage of dual-sensor or multiple-sensor systems over a single sensor is not yet certain, and likely varies depending on specific patient cohorts. The advantage of dual-/multiple-sensor pacing is more likely to be obtained in patients with an active lifestyle. Whether the complexity of such systems (ie, requiring more attention to programming) and their added cost outweigh any physiologic benefit are questions that are not likely to be resolved for some time.

Technology for sensors in heart-failure patients with cardiac implantable electronic devices continues to evolve. Many diagnostic parameters can be monitored by implanted devices, although the clinical utility of such monitoring remains to be determined. In particular, hemodynamic sensors may play an important role in the long-term monitoring of and early intervention in patients with heart failure, especially if methods evolve to permit reliable assessment of the key hemodynamic variables (preload, afterload, left ventricular ejection fraction, and stroke volume).

REFERENCES

1. Cammilli L, Alcidi L, Papeschi G. A new pacemaker autoregulating the rate of pacing in relation to metabolic needs. Amsterdam: Excerpta Medica; 1976.

2. Benditt DG, Mianulli M, Lurie K, et al. Multiple-sensor systems for physiologic cardiac pacing. Ann Intern Med 1994;121:960–8.

3. Benditt DG, Mianulli M, Fetter J, et al. Single-chamber cardiac pacing with activity-initiated chronotropic response: evaluation by cardiopulmonary exercise testing. Circulation 1987;7:184–91.

4. Rossi P. Rate-responsive pacing: biosensor reliability and physiological sensitivity. Pacing Clin Electrophysiol 1987;10(3 Pt 1):454–66.

5. Lau CP, Antoniou A, Ward DE, et al. Initial clinical experience with a minute ventilation sensing rate modulated pacemaker: improvements in exercise capacity and symptomatology. Pacing Clin Electrophysiol 1988;11(11 Pt 2):1815–22.

6. Mond H, Strathmore N, Kertes P, et al. Rate responsive pacing using a minute ventilation sensor. Pacing Clin Electrophysiol 1988;11(11 Pt 2):1866–74.

7. Rossi P, Plicchi G, Canducci G, et al. Respiratory rate as a determinant of optimal pacing rate. Pacing Clin Electrophysiol 1983;6(2 Pt 2):502–10.

8. Wirtzfeld A, Goedel-Meinen L, Bock T, et al. Central venous oxygen saturation for the control of automatic rate-responsive pacing. Pacing Clin Electrophysiol 1982;5:829–35.

9. Rickards AF, Norman J. Relation between QT interval and heart rate. New design of physiologically adaptive cardiac pacemaker. Br Heart J 1981;45:56–61.

10. Cammilli L. Initial use of a pH triggered pacemaker. Pacing Clin Electrophysiol 1989;12:1000–7.

11. Alt E, Matula M, Theres H, et al. The basis for activity controlled rate variable cardiac pacemakers: an analysis of mechanical forces on the human body induced by exercise and environment. Pacing Clin Electrophysiol 1989;12:1667–80.

12. Fetter J, Benditt DG, Mianulli M. Usefulness of transcutaneous triggering of conventional implanted pulse generators by an activity-sensing pacemaker for predicting effectiveness of rate response pacing. Am J Cardiol 1988;62:901–5.

13. Benditt DG, Mianulli M, Fetter J, et al. An office-based exercise protocol for predicting chronotropic response of activity-triggered, rate-variable pacemakers. Am J Cardiol 1989;64:27–32.

14. Anderson KM, Moore AA. Sensors in pacing. Pacing Clin Electrophysiol 1986;9(6 Pt 2):954–9.

15. Schmidt M, Ammer R, Evans F, et al. Improving accelerometer-based rate adaptive pacing by means of second-generation signal processing. Pacing Clin Electrophysiol 1996;19(11 Pt 2):1698–703.

16. Menozzi C, Brignole M, Moracchini PV, et al. Intra-patient comparison between chronic VVIR and DDD pacing in patients affected by high degree AV block without heart failure. Pacing Clin Electrophysiol 1990;13(12 Pt 2):1816–22.

17. Oldroyd KG, Rae AP, Carter R, et al. Double blind crossover comparison of the effects of dual chamber pacing (DDD) and ventricular rate adaptive (VVIR) pacing on neuroendocrine variables, exercise performance, and symptoms in complete heart block. Br Heart J 1991;65:188–93.

18. Candinas R, Jakob M, Buckingham TA, et al. Vibration, acceleration, gravitation, and movement: activity controlled rate adaptive pacing during treadmill exercise testing and daily life activities. Pacing Clin Electrophysiol 1997;20:1777–86.

19. Alt E, Matula M, Holzer K. Behavior of different activity-based pacemakers during treadmill exercise testing with variable slopes: a comparison of three activity-based pacing systems. Pacing Clin Electrophysiol 1994;17(11 Pt 1):1761–70.

20. Shukla HH, Flaker GC, Hellkamp AS, et al. Clinical and quality of life comparison of accelerometer, piezoelectric crystal, and blended sensors in DDDR-paced patients with sinus node dysfunction in the mode selection trial (MOST). Pacing Clin Electrophysiol 2005;28:762–70.

21. Coman J, Freedman R, Koplan BA, et al. A blended sensor restores chronotropic response more favorably than an accelerometer alone in pacemaker patients: the LIFE study results. Pacing Clin Electrophysiol 2008;31:1433–42.

22. Whellan DJ, Ousdigian KT, Al-Khatib SM, et al. Combined heart failure device diagnostics identify patients at higher risk of subsequent heart failure hospitalizations: results from PARTNERS HF (Program to Access and Review Trending Information and Evaluate Correlation to Symptoms in Patients with Heart Failure) study. J Am Coll Cardiol 2010;55(17):1803–10.

23. Kubisch K, Peters W, Chiladakis I, et al. Clinical experience with the rate responsive pacemaker Sensolog 703. Pacing Clin Electrophysiol 1988;11(11 Pt 2):1829–33.

24. Candinas RA, Gloor HO, Amann FW, et al. Activity-sensing rate responsive versus conventional fixed-rate pacing: a comparison of rate behavior and patient well-being during routine daily exercise. Pacing Clin Electrophysiol 1991;14(2 Pt 1):204–13.

25. Matula M, Schlegl M, Alt E. Activity controlled cardiac pacemakers during stairwalking: a comparison of accelerometer with vibration guided devices and with sinus rate. Pacing Clin Electrophysiol 1996;19:1036–41.

26. Lau CP, Mehta D, Toff WD, et al. Limitations of rate response of an activity-sensing rate-responsive pacemaker to different forms of activity. Pacing Clin Electrophysiol 1988;11:141–50.

27. Vai F, Bonnet JL, Ritter P, et al. Relationship between heart rate and minute ventilation, tidal volume and respiratory rate during brief and low level exercise. Pacing Clin Electrophysiol 1988; 11(11 Pt 2):1860–5.

28. Duru F, Cho Y, Wilkoff BL, et al. Rate responsive pacing using transthoracic impedance minute ventilation sensors: a multicenter study on calibration stability. Pacing Clin Electrophysiol 2002;25: 1679–84.

29. Hauser RG. Techniques for improving cardiac performance with implantable devices. Pacing Clin Electrophysiol 1984;7(6 Pt 2):1234–9.

30. Osswald S, Cron T, Gradel C, et al. Closed-loop stimulation using intracardiac impedance as a sensor principle: correlation of right ventricular dP/dtmax and intracardiac impedance during dobutamine stress test. Pacing Clin Electrophysiol 2000;23(10 Pt 1):1502–8.

31. Occhetta E, Bortnik M, Audoglio R, et al. Closed loop stimulation in prevention of vasovagal syncope. Inotropy Controlled Pacing in Vasovagal Syncope (INVASY): a multicentre randomized, single blind, controlled study. Europace 2004;6: 538–47.

32. Langenfeld H, Krein A, Kirstein M, et al. Peak endocardial acceleration-based clinical testing of the "BEST" DDDR pacemaker. European PEA Clinical Investigation Group. Pacing Clin Electrophysiol 1998;21(11 Pt 2):2187–91.

33. Clementy J. Dual chamber rate responsive pacing system driven by contractility: final assessment after 1-year follow-up. The European PEA Clinical Investigation Group. Pacing Clin Electrophysiol 1998;21(11 Pt 2):2192–7.

34. Deharo JC, Brunetto AB, Bellocci F, et al. DDDR pacing driven by contractility versus DDI pacing in vasovagal syncope: a multicenter, randomized study. Pacing Clin Electrophysiol 2003;26(1 Pt 2): 447–50.

35. Delnoy PP, Marcelli E, Oudeluttikhuis H, et al. Validation of a peak endocardial acceleration-based algorithm to optimize cardiac resynchronization: early clinical results. Europace 2008;10:801–8.

36. Alt E, Hirgstetter C, Heinz M, et al. Rate control of physiologic pacemakers by central venous blood temperature. Circulation 1986;73:1206–12.

37. Lau CP, Wong CK, Leung WH, et al. A comparative evaluation of a minute ventilation sensing and activity sensing adaptive-rate pacemakers during daily activities. Pacing Clin Electrophysiol 1989; 12:1514–21.

38. Lau CP, Butrous GS, Ward DE, et al. Comparison of exercise performance of six rate-adaptive right ventricular cardiac pacemakers. Am J Cardiol 1989;63(12):833–8.

39. Leung SK, Lau CP, Wu CW, et al. Quantitative comparison of rate response and oxygen uptake kinetics between different sensor modes in multisensor rate adaptive pacing. Pacing Clin Electrophysiol 1994;17(11 Pt 2):1920–7.

40. Connelly DT. Initial experience with a new single chamber, dual sensor rate responsive pacemaker. The Topaz Study Group. Pacing Clin Electrophysiol 1993;16:1833–41.

41. Leung SK, Lau CP, Tang MO. Cardiac output is a sensitive indicator of difference in exercise performance between single and dual sensor pacemakers. Pacing Clin Electrophysiol 1998;21(1 Pt 1): 35–41.

42. Leung SK, Lau CP, Tang MO, et al. New integrated sensor pacemaker: comparison of rate responses between an integrated minute ventilation and activity sensor and single sensor modes during exercise and daily activities and nonphysiological interference. Pacing Clin Electrophysiol 1996; 19(11 Pt 2):1664–71.

43. Lau CP, Rushby J, Leigh-Jones M, et al. Symptomatology and quality of life in patients with rate-responsive pacemakers: a double-blind, randomized, crossover study. Clin Cardiol 1989; 12(9):505–12.

44. Lau CP, Tai YT, Leung WH, et al. Rate adaptive pacing in sick sinus syndrome: effects of pacing modes and intrinsic conduction on physiological responses, arrhythmias, symptomatology and quality of life. Eur Heart J 1994;15(11):1445–55.

45. Nielsen JC, Thomsen PE, Hojberg S, et al. A comparison of single-lead atrial pacing with dual-chamber pacing in sick sinus syndrome. Eur Heart J 2011;32(6):686–96.

46. Lamas GA, Knight JD, Sweeney MO, et al. Impact of rate-modulated pacing on quality of life and exercise capacity–evidence from the Advanced Elements of Pacing Randomized Controlled Trial (ADEPT). Heart Rhythm 2007;4(9):1125–32.

47. Tse HF, Wong KK, Siu CW, et al. Upgrading pacemaker patients with right ventricular apical pacing to right ventricular septal pacing improves left ventricular performance and functional capacity. J Cardiovasc Electrophysiol 2009;20(8): 901–5.

48. Plicchi G, Marcelli E, Parlapiano M, et al. PEA I and PEA II based implantable haemodynamic monitor: pre-clinical studies in sheep. Europace 2002;4(1): 49–54.

49. Gras D, Kubler L, Ritter P, et al. Recording of peak endocardial acceleration in the atrium. Pacing Clin Electrophysiol 2009;32(Suppl 1):S240–6.

50. Yu CM, Wang L, Chau E, et al. Intrathoracic impedance monitoring in patients with heart failure: correlation with fluid status and feasibility of early

warning preceding hospitalization. Circulation 2005;112(6):841–8.

51. Catanzariti D, Lunati M, Landolina M, et al. Monitoring intrathoracic impedance with an implantable defibrillator reduces hospitalizations in patients with heart failure. Pacing Clin Electrophysiol 2009; 32(3):363–70.

52. Abraham WT, Compton S, Haas G, et al. Intrathoracic impedance vs daily weight monitoring for predicting worsening heart failure events: results of the Fluid Accumulation Status Trial (FAST). Congest Heart Fail 2011;17(2):51–5.

53. Kaye G, Arthur W, Edgar D, et al. The use of unipolar intracardiac impedance for discrimination of haemodynamically stable and unstable arrhythmias in man. Europace 2006;8(11):988–93.

54. Stahl C, Beierlein W, Walker T, et al. Intracardiac impedance monitors hemodynamic deterioration in a chronic heart failure pig model. J Cardiovasc Electrophysiol 2007;18(9):985–90.

55. Bocchiardo M, Meyer zu Vilsendorf D, Militello C, et al. Intracardiac impedance monitors stroke volume in resynchronization therapy patients. Europace 2010;12(5):702–7.

Advanced Sensors for ICDs

Zhongwei Cheng, MD[a], Paul J. Wang, MD, FHRS[b],*

KEYWORDS

- Implantable cardioverter defibrillator • Heart rate variability • Pulmonary artery pressure
- Left atrial pressure • Intrathoracic impedance • Myocardial ischemia monitoring

KEY POINTS

- Sensors may assess physical activity, heart rate variability, thoracic impedance, and myocardial ischemia.
- Intracardiac monitoring of right ventricular systolic pulmonary artery pressure and left atrial pressure has promise in guiding therapy in the future.
- Monitoring sensors might permit interventions to prevent heart failure and heart failure hospitalization and to detect early myocardial ischemia.

INTRODUCTION

Implantable cardioverter defibrillators (ICDs) have become a standard part of the treatment of patients at risk for life-threatening ventricular arrhythmias. These devices are capable of capturing more and more data that may aid in patient management. Most devices have remote monitoring capabilities that further assist in providing important clinical data at all times. Sensor data represent critical information for patient management, in addition to battery status, arrhythmic events, and lead information. Because many patients with ICDs have heart failure (HF) and/or a risk for coronary artery disease, hemodynamic and ischemia monitoring may be particularly important. Use of cardiac resynchronization therapy (CRT) further increases the need for sensor information in patient management. There are numerous types of sensors that are available, being developed, or in clinical investigation (**Table 1**). This review focuses on sensors that may be useful for patient management in patients with ICDs with, and without, resynchronization therapy.

HEART RATE AND ACTIVITY SENSORS
Physical Activity

Physical activity can be assessed using accelerometers, which measure acceleration within space. Because physical activity may be an indicator of the patient's overall degree of physical functioning, measurements of changes in activity may alert the clinician to changes in the patient's health condition. For some patients, these changes may reflect alterations in cardiovascular status, but for others there may be additional causes of lack of activity. Using the accelerometer data, a mean daily physical activity index can be calculated to measure the time in minutes per day with physical activity greater than 70 steps per minute walk rate. Braunschweig and colleagues[1] showed that changes in physical activity could reflect the improvement of HF status. A total of 56 patients with New York Heart Association (NYHA) functional class II to IV, with implanted CRT devices, were included in the prospective, nonrandomized InSync III Study. The activity trend over 3 months was significantly greater in patients

Disclosures: Dr Wang has received honoraria from Boston Scientific and Medtronic, Inc.
a Department of Cardiology, Peking Union Medical College Hospital, Peking Union Medical College and Chinese Academy of Medical Sciences, No. 1 Shuaifuyuan, Wangfujing, Dongcheng District, Beijing 100730, China; b Cardiovascular Medicine, Stanford University, 300 Pasteur Drive, Suite H 2146, Stanford, CA 94305, USA
* Corresponding author.
E-mail address: pjwang@stanford.edu

Table 1
Sensor parameters categorized by availability or investigational status

Parameter	In Investigation/Available
Body motion	Available
Activity	Available
Lead acceleration	Available
Temperature	Not available
Heart rate variability	Available
Thoracic impedance	Available
Pulmonary artery pressure	In investigation
Left atrial pressure	In investigation
ECG ischemia	Available
Autonomic sensor	Not available

with better functional status at baseline. During the first 4 weeks of treatment, activity increased significantly in all patient groups, as defined by NYHA classification.

Heart Rate Variability

A variety of algorithms have been used to assess changes in autonomic function. Heart rate variability (HRV) is the most commonly used measurement to assess the body's autonomic function. Autonomic and neurohormonal systems are critical in meeting the physiologic demands of the body, in both the presence and the absence of HF.

HF patients exhibit decreased HRV, indicating autonomic dysfunction. HRV had been measured using several methods, including Holter monitoring. Heart rate control is under the influence of sympathetic and parasympathetic innervation at the sinoatrial node.[2] Vagal input results in high-frequency cyclic fluctuations in heart rate,

and sympathetic stimulation results in a low-frequency effect on heart rate, eventually reducing HRV. The circadian changes in heart rate during the day and night are also mediated through a complex neurohormonal mechanism including the renin-angiotensin system.[3] With increased physiologic stress such as HF exacerbation, there is an increase in heart rate variability due to an increase in sympathetic input and/or parasympathetic withdrawal. Several studies have demonstrated that heart rate variability is a predictor of mortality after myocardial infarction and in the presence of HF.[4–7]

The standard deviation of measured Normal Sinus to Normal Sinus (NN) interval over a period of time is a commonly used time domain measure of HRV. The standard deviation of average intrinsic interval over 5 minutes (SDANN)[7] and the standard deviation of the 5-minute median A-A interval[8] are 2 examples of such measurements and can be derived from measurements in ICDs. One display of heart variability as it changes with sinus rate is the HRV footprint available in some Boston Scientific ICDs (Natick, MA, USA). During a 24-hour period, the intrinsic sinus rate is shown on the x-axis and the HRV is shown on the y-axis. The frequency (third dimension) of each heart rate and variability occurrence is indicated by color (where red and orange indicate more frequent and blue and gray indicate less frequent).[9] Increased size of HRV footprint showed decreased mortality risk. **Fig. 1** shows the HRV footprint of a 65-year-old CRT-D patient, who had an HRV of 24% at pre-discharge and an HRV of 76% at 6 months after CRT-D. The SDANN and HRV footprint can be automatically evaluated and stored by the CRT-D device at each device interrogation.

Decreased HRV and high mean heart rates in patients with HF are associated with poor prognosis[10,11] and previous β-blocker trials have demonstrated that the HRV and the mean heart

A

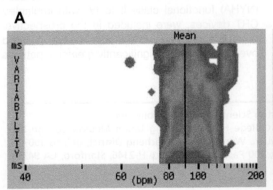

B

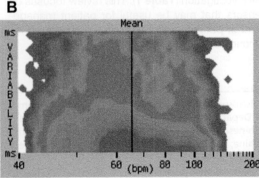

Fig. 1. HRV footprint of a 65-year-old CRT-D patient. The HRV footprint was 24% at pre-discharge check (*A*) and increased to 76% at the checkup 6 months after CRT-D implantation (*B*).

rates improved with treatment and were associated with improved prognosis.[12] In addition, daily activity levels measured were predictive of mortality.[13] Because ICDs have the ability to measure heart rate variability, activity, and mean heart rates, it is important to determine if ICD data could predict mortality and outcome.

Gilliam and colleagues[14] showed that continuously measured device-based HRV parameters (SDANN and HRV footprint) could provide prognostic information and might be helpful for risk stratification. A total of 842 patients (age, 67.7 ± 11.2; 23.5% female; NYHA class III, 88.6%; class IV, 11.4%) with implanted CRT-D devices were included. During a median of 11.6 months of follow-up, 7.8% (66/842) of patients died. HRV footprint and SDANN were significant predictors of mortality (all P<.05); patients with lower HRV values were at greater risk for death, compared with patients with higher HRV values. HRV changes over time tended to predict the risk of mortality in follow-up; patients with low baseline HRV and small changes in HRV during the follow-up period were at the highest risk for death (7% mortality for SDANN and 8.9% for HRV footprint), and patients with high baseline HRV and large changes in HRV were at the lowest risk (1.5% mortality for SDANN and 2.4% for HRV footprint). The HF-HRV registry is the largest study to date to assess the relationship between CRT-D measured HRV parameters and outcomes.[15] The study results demonstrated that CRT-D devices were able to measure the changes of HRV parameters significantly associated with improved patient outcomes. The registry enrolled 1421 patients with implanted CRT-D devices capable of measuring HRV parameters, including SDANN and HRV footprint. The study showed an overall improvement in SDANN (69.2 ± 25.5, 78.5 ± 27.8, 79.4 ± 27.2, 80.7 ± 28.2) and HRV footprint (31.5 ± 11.8, 33.4 ± 12.3, 34.2 ± 12.2, 34.5 ± 12.3) at the 2-week, 3-month, 6-month, and 12-month visits, respectively (both P<.001). There were also significant changes over time in clinical status (improved quality of life, increased activity, and improved NYHA, all P<.0001).

ICD diagnostics have been used to create a model to predict mortality. Singh and colleagues[16] examined 2 CRT studies, the Cardiac Resynchronization Therapy Registry Evaluating Patient Response with RENEWAL Family Devices (CRT RENEWAL) (n = 436) and HF-HRV registry (n = 838). Patients from CRT RENEWAL were used to create a model for risk of death using logistic regression and to create a scoring system (each patient received either 0 or 1 for the absence or presence of the following diagnostics at the 2-week visit: SDANN <43, mean HR >74, footprint <29, and activity percent >5; low risk was score of 0–1, moderate risk was score of 2–3, high risk was score of 3–4) that could be used to predict mortality. Both were validated in a cohort of patients from the HF-HRV registry. Diagnostics significantly improved over time post-CRT implant (all P<.001) and correlated with a trend of decreased risk of death. The regression model classified CRT RENEWAL patients into low (2.8%), moderate (6.9%), and high (13.8%) risk of death based on tertiles of their model predicted risk. The clinical risk score classified CRT RENEWAL patients into low (2.8%), moderate (10.1%), and high (13.4%) risk of death based on tertiles of their score. When the regression model and the clinical risk score were applied to the HF-HRV registry, each was able to classify patients into appropriate levels of risk. **Fig. 2** shows a Kaplan–Meier curve for HF-HRV registry of time to death by clinical scoring system grouping.

HRV is influenced by a wide variety of factors, including medications, diabetes status, sleeping patterns, smoking status, and renal disease[17–20] and varies considerably over time. Therefore, its role in preventing hospitalization is still not clear and its predictability for HF exacerbation in comparison to other established parameters remains undetermined.

INTRATHORACIC IMPEDANCE MONITORING

A high-frequency electrical current passed between the device case (typically implanted in the left pectoral region) and a lead in the right ventricle may be used to measure the opposition to current flow across the chest, a parameter called thoracic impedance (TI). Accumulation of intrathoracic fluid in pulmonary edema results in a decrease in the TI. Animal studies[21] showed that the changes of impedance, measured by the implanted devices with right ventricular leads, had a strong inverse correlation with changes of directly measured extravascular lung water index and changes in the LV end-diastolic pressure.[22]

Several studies have demonstrated the ability of OptiVol index (OI; Medtronic, Minneapolis, MN, USA) Medtronic's approach to impedance monitoring, to estimate TI in humans. The Medtronic Impedance Diagnostics in Heart Failure Patients Trial[23] was the first clinical trial to assess the efficacy of OptiVol fluid status monitor. Although relatively small in sample size, the study demonstrated the possibility of providing an advanced warning of pulmonary congestion at a presymptomatic stage and enabling early interventions with the goal of preventing HF exacerbation. Ypenburg

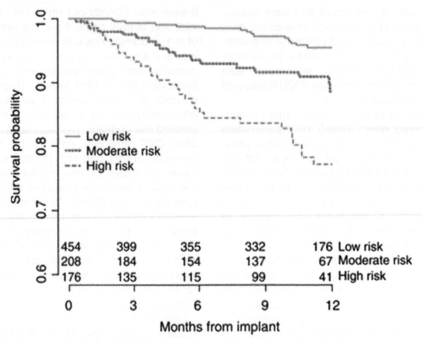

Fig. 2. The Kaplan–Meier curve for HF-HRV registry of time to death by clinical scoring system grouping. (*From* Singh JP, Rosenthal LS, Hranitzky PM, et al. Device diagnostics and long-term clinical outcome in patients receiving cardiac resynchronization therapy. Europace 2009;11:1647–53; with permission.)

and colleagues[24] reported that OptiVol fluid status monitor might be a useful tool for monitoring pulmonary fluid status and predicting HF exacerbation. One hundred fifteen consecutive patients, mean NYHA class 2.8 ± 0.5, mean ejection fraction 26 ± 8%, had a CRT-D device implanted. A total of 45 presentations with OptiVol alert in 30 patients occurred during 9 ± 5 months of follow-up. The results showed that increasing the threshold for the OptiVol alert provided a substantial increase in specificity for the detection of HF, with the optimal cutoff value identified at 120 Ω/day, yielding a sensitivity of 60% and specificity of 73%. Maines and colleagues[25] showed that the OptiVol fluid status monitor was a useful tool in reducing hospitalization in HF patients in a case-control study. The 2 groups had similar clinical characteristics, each group consisting of 27 consecutive patients implanted with CRT-D devices. Group 1 was with the OptiVol fluid status monitor feature turned on and group 2 was not. In group 1, 12 of the 27 patients experienced 18 OptiVol alarms with only one hospital admission during the follow-up of 359 ± 98 days. In group 2, eight HF hospitalizations occurred in 7 patients (P<.05). The results showed that the OptiVol fluid status monitor feature was a useful tool for early treatment during the preclinical stage of HF exacerbation and resulted in a significant reduction of hospital admissions. Jhanjee and colleagues[26]

showed that worsening pulmonary congestion assessed by OI was associated with increased atrial tachyarrhythmia frequency in patients with left ventricular dysfunction. A total of 59 patients (mean left ventricular ejection fraction, 24%) with implanted OI-capable ICDs with 225 follow-up visits (mean, 3.8 visits per patient) were retrospectively studied. The OI values were stratified into 3 levels: group 1, <40; group 2, 40 to 60; and group 3, >60. Atrial tachyarrhythmia frequency was greater in group 3 versus group 1 (P = .0342). Moore and colleagues[27] reported that decreased TI preceded ventricular tachycardia/fibrillation (VT/VF) episodes. A total of 317 VT/VF episodes in a cohort of 121 patients with implanted OptiVol-capable ICDs were retrospectively studied. Average daily TI decreased preceding 64% of VT/VF episodes, with an average decrease of 0.46 ± 0.35 Ω on the day before the VT/VF episodes. A novel measure, ΔTI, the sum of the daily differences between the averaged daily and reference impedance, was negative preceding 66% of VT/VF episodes (P<.001). Ip and colleagues[28] reported that in HF patients who developed VT/VF, volume overload, assessed by TI, was temporally associated with malignant ventricular tachyarrhythmias. A cohort of 96 patients with left ventricular dysfunction (ejection fraction ≤35%) with implanted OptiVol-capable devices was studied. VT/VF episodes occurred in 16 patients (17%).

VT/VF was more common on days when the fluid index was elevated using predetermined threshold values of 15, 30, and 45 Ω/days (P = .006, .04, .02, respectively). Maines and colleagues[29] reported that the changes in ICD-measured impedance seemed associated with the LV volume changes induced by CRT-D, especially the LV-to-RV impedance. A total of 170 patients with implanted OptiVol-capable CRT-D devices were studied. LV end-systolic volume decreased at 6-month follow-up (vs baseline, group A) in 127 patients and the remaining 43 patients (group B) had a change $\geq$0. The impedances of groups A and B gradually diverged soon after the implant, resulting in a significant difference between the 2 groups at the 6-month visit (P = .001). The changes in LV dimensions produced larger differences between groups in the impedance measured between the LV and the RV leads (P<.001). The regression analysis demonstrated an inverse correlation between paired changes of volume and TI. 3D-HF (Diagnostic Data for Discharge in Heart Failure Patients) study[30] was a prospective observational pilot study enrolling HF patients with OptiVol-capable devices who were admitted because of worsening HF symptoms. The primary end point was the difference in times from admission to 50% improvement in impedance and to when the patient was medically ready for discharge. A total of 20 patients were enrolled, and the median length of stay was 7 days. Eighteen patients achieved the TI improvement before discharge. The time to reach the threshold for improvement was 2.5 days. The study showed that OptiVol fluid monitor could be used as a tool and a potential criterion for discharge readiness for patients admitted for acute HF exacerbation.

Several other factors influence the TI, including skin and muscle within the electric field of concern, pleural effusion, air volume in the lung, trauma, infection, and pregnancy,[31,32] explaining the low reproducibility of TI measurement. Any pulmonary events that occur in the lung contralateral to the implanted device should not affect the intrathoracic impedance data. Therefore, consideration should be given for those diseases or conditions that might affect the TI measurements. A recent study about OptiVol fluid status monitoring demonstrated inconsistent results with previous studies. van Veldhuisen and colleagues[33] on behalf of DOT-HF Investigators reported that measuring TI with an audible patient alert did not improve outcome and increased HF hospitalizations and outpatient visits in HF patients. A total of 335 chronic HF patients with implanted OptiVol-capable ICD (18%) or CRT-D (82%) were randomized to have information available to physicians and patients as an audible alert in cases of preset threshold crossings (access arm) or not (control arm). The primary end point was a composite of all-cause mortality and HF hospitalizations. During the follow-up of 14.9 ± 5.4 months, the primary end point occurred in 48 patients (29%) in the access arm and in 33 patients (20%) in the control arm (P = .063), due mainly to more HF hospitalizations (P = .022), whereas the number of deaths was comparable (P = .54). The number of outpatient visits was higher in the access arm (250 vs 84; P<.0001). Therefore, further studies are needed to clarify whether fluid status monitoring with OptiVol-capable ICDs could reduce cardiovascular-related hospitalizations and mortality in HF patients. The Optimization of Heart Failure Management using OptiVol Fluid Status Monitoring and CareLink (OptiLink HF) study,[34] designed to investigate whether OptiVol fluid status monitoring with an automatically generated wireless CareAlert notification via the CareLink Network can reduce all-cause death and cardiovascular hospitalizations in an HF population, compared with standard clinical assessment, is ongoing. The first study results are expected to be reported in May 2014.

INTRACARDIAC HEMODYNAMIC MONITORING

The measurement of intracardiac pressures has been an important part of the invasive assessment of the HF patient. Incorporation of sensors capable of measuring intracardiac pressures into ICDs might contribute significantly to the management of HF. An implantable device capable of measuring right ventricular pressure has been studied clinically. Zile and colleagues[35] examined patients with class III/IV HF in the COMPASS-III study. The RV pressure measured at the time of pulmonary valve opening has been strongly correlated with the pulmonary artery diastolic pressure.

In systolic HF and diastolic HF patients who developed acute decompensated HF, these events were associated with a significant increase in estimated pulmonary artery diastolic pressure (ePAD), from 17 ± to 22 ± 7 mm (P<.05) in diastolic heart failure patients and from 21 ± 9 to 24 ± 8 mm Hg (P<.05) in systolic heart failure patients.

By using a novel lead with an encapsulated pressure transducer inserted into the atrial septum, it is possible to obtain left atrial pressure measurements. A hand-held device is used to obtain pressure data from the implanted sensor and to power the sensor using a 128-kHz radiofrequency electromagnetic induction. Pressure drift did not exceed 1.3 mm Hg at any quarterly measurement. Freedom from device failure was 95% at 2 years.

The measurements from the device correlated well with invasively obtained measurements of pulmonary capillary wedge pressure (r = 0.92; difference 1.1 ± 3.9 mm Hg).[36]

MYOCARDIAL ISCHEMIA MONITORING (ST-SEGMENT MONITORING)

It is well-established that ICDs prevent sudden cardiac death. The progression of the underlying heart disease became the prime determinant of the patient's prognosis. In most ICD implanted patients suffering from coronary artery disease, such progression is characterized by new-onset ischemia, acute myocardial infarction, and/or the development of ischemic cardiomyopathy. Myocardial ischemia monitoring by the ICDs would therefore provide an interesting new diagnostic option in these patients. New-onset ischemia, any change in the frequency, and severity of ischemic episodes, as well as the patient's daily ischemic burden would become routinely assessable whenever necessary. The intracardiac electrocardiogram (IT-ECG) leads derived from presently available electrodes in ICDs (located in the right ventricle, the superior vena cava [SVC], and at the generator site) might provide the structural basis for monitoring ischemia in ICD patients. Because of these considerations, continuous ICD monitoring of myocardial ischemia could markedly increase the diagnostic impact of this device.[37,38] Currently, the most simple and reliable technique for monitoring ischemia is based on the ST-segment analysis. Algorithms directed to the assessment of ischemic ST-segment changes have been developed.[38,39]

An animal study[40] showed that an implantable ischemia detection system (IIDS) with real-time alerting capability to detect ST-segment elevation from coronary occlusion was feasible. All 8 stented pigs had acute ST-segment elevation events triggering the alerting thresholds of the IIDS. Four of the 8 pigs died of VF, recorded by the IIDS at

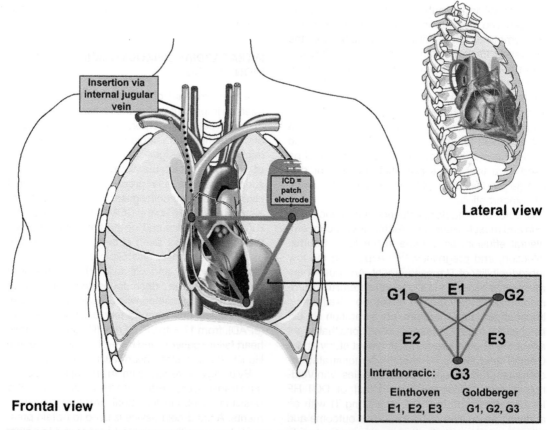

Fig. 3. The illustration of 6 IT-ECG leads (according to Einthoven, E1–E3 and Goldberger, G1–G3) by use of 3 electrodes placed in the RVA and SVA (inserted via the internal jugular vein) and the generator site (cutaneous patch). (*From* Baron TW, Faber TS, Grom A, et al. Real-time assessment of acute myocardial ischaemia by an intra-thoracic 6-lead ECG: evaluation of a new diagnostic option in the implantable defibrillator. Europace 2006;8:996; with permission).

a mean time of 70 ± 121 hours after ST-segment alert. The sensitivity and specificity of alerting for ST-segment shift, associated with thrombotic coronary occlusion, were 100% and 100%, respectively. Another animal study[41] showed that intrathoracic far-field electrocardiograms (FF-ECG) could provide reliable and reproducible detection of experimentally induced ischemia originating from all major coronary arteries. In 7 pigs with an ICD implanted in the left pectoral region and electrodes placed in the right ventricle and the SVC, all major coronary arteries in proximal and distal locations were occluded for 180 seconds each. Reliable detection of ischemia by ST-segment analysis was possible in all (38/38) experiments. Maximum deviation from baseline was larger in FF-ECG (1.21 mV) than surface ECG leads (0.23 mV, $P<.01$) for all occlusion sites. Ischemia could be detected earlier ($P<.05$) in the FF-ECG, with a sensitivity of 100%, 93%, and 100% after occlusions in the left anterior descending, left circumflex, and right coronary arteries, respectively. Baron and colleagues[42] showed that ICD-based intrathoracic 6-lead ECG could provide a new and efficient means of assessing a patient's daily ischemic burden. In 22 patients undergoing percutaneous transluminal coronary angioplasty, 3 electrodes, similar to those used in the ICD, were inserted to create 6 IT-ECG leads according to Einthoven and Goldberger. The diagnostic efficacy for ischemia assessment was compared with the surface ECG. The IT-ECG proved to be more sensitive than conventional ECG in early and overall ischemia assessment. Intrathoracic Einthoven 2 (Superior vena cava + Right ventricular apex vs ICD-housing) and Goldberger 3 (Superior vena cava + ICD-housing vs Right ventricular apex) had the highest sensitivity (88/85%). The 6 IT-ECG leads (according to Einthoven, E1–E3 and Goldberger, G1–G3) by use of 3 electrodes placed in the RVA and SVA (inserted via the internal jugular vein) and the generator site (cutaneous patch) are illustrated in **Fig. 3**.

However, a recent study[43] showed that ICD-based ST-segment monitoring failed to provide a benefit over ICDs without this capability and increased unscheduled evaluations in patients with remote follow-up. This was a prospective, controlled, and nonrandomized study with patients implanted with ICDs with continuous intracardiac ST-segment monitoring (ST group, n = 53) or without (n = 50). During 15.4 ± 8.4 months of follow-up, one patient experienced ST-segment shift events, which was confirmed by angiography to be related to myocardial ischemia. In the ST group, 7 patients had ≥1 episodes of false-positive ST-segment events (median 9,

range 1–90). Among patients with a remote monitoring system, unscheduled outpatient visits were significantly increased in the ST group (17 vs 4; $P = .032$).

SUMMARY

Sensors that reflect physical activity, HRV, TI, and myocardial ischemia monitoring may add importantly to the capabilities of ICDs in patient management. Intracardiac monitoring of RV systolic pulmonary artery pressure and left atrial pressure exhibits considerable promise in guiding therapy in the future. Monitoring these sensors might allow appropriate interventions to prevent HF and HF hospitalization and to detect early myocardial ischemia.

REFERENCES

1. Braunschweig F, Mortensen PT, Gras D, et al, InSync III Study Investigators. Monitoring of physical activity and heart rate variability in patients with chronic heart failure using cardiac resynchronization devices. Am J Cardiol 2005;95:1104–7.
2. Lombardi F. Clinical implications of present physiological understanding of HRV components. Card Electrophysiol Rev 2002;6:245–9.
3. Molgaard H, Sorensen KE, Bjerregaard P. Circadian variation and influence of risk factors on heart rate variability in healthy subjects. Am J Cardiol 1991; 68:777–84.
4. Malik M, Camm AJ, Janse MJ, et al. Depressed heart rate variability identifies postinfarction patients who might benefit from prophylactic treatment with amiodarone: a substudy of EMIAT (The European Myocardial Infarct Amiodarone Trial). J Am Coll Cardiol 2000;35:1263–75.
5. Adamson PB, Vanoli E. Early autonomic and repolarization abnormalities contribute to lethal arrhythmias in chronic ischemic heart failure: characteristics of a novel heart failure model in dogs with post myocardial infarction left ventricular dysfunction. J Am Coll Cardiol 2001;37:1741–8.
6. La Rovere MT, Pinna GD, Hohnloser SH, et al, ATRAMI Investigators. Autonomic Tone and Reflexes After Myocardial Infarcton. Baroreflex sensitivity and heart rate variability in the identification of patients at risk for life-threatening arrhythmias: implications for clinical trials. Circulation 2001;103:2072–7.
7. Fantoni C, Raffa S, Regoli F, et al. Cardiac resynchronization therapy improves heart rate profile and heart rate variability of patients with moderate to severe heart failure. J Am Coll Cardiol 2005;46: 1875–82.
8. Adamson PB, Smith AL, Abraham WT, et al, InSync III Model 8042 and Attain OTW Lead Model 4193 Clinical

Trial Investigators. Continuous autonomic assessment in patients with symptomatic heart failure: prognostic value of heart rate variability measured by an implanted cardiac resynchronization device. Circulation 2004;110:2389–94.

9. Carlson G, Girouard S, Schlegl M, et al. Three-dimensional heart rate variability diagnostic for monitoring heart failure through an implantable device. J Cardiovasc Electrophysiol 2004;15:506.

10. Nolan J, Batin PD, Andrews R, et al. Prospective study of heart rate variability and mortality in chronic heart failure: results of the United Kingdom heart failure evaluation and assessment of risk trial (UK HEART). Circulation 1998;98:1510–6.

11. La Rovere MT, Pinna GD, Maestri R, et al. Short-term heart rate variability strongly predicts sudden cardiac death in chronic heart failure patients. Circulation 2003;107:565–70.

12. Mortara A, La Rovere MT, Pinna GD, et al. Nonselective beta-adrenergic blocking agent, carvedilol, improves arterial baroreflex gain and heart rate variability in patients with stable chronic heart failure. J Am Coll Cardiol 2000;36:1612–8.

13. Walsh JT, Charlesworth A, Andrews R, et al. Relation of daily activity levels in patients with chronic heart failure to long-term prognosis. Am J Cardiol 1997;79:1364–9.

14. Gilliam FR 3rd, Singh JP, Mullin CM, et al. Prognostic value of heart rate variability footprint and standard deviation of average 5-minute intrinsic R-R intervals for mortality in cardiac resynchronization therapy patients. J Electrocardiol 2007;40:336–42.

15. Gilliam FR 3rd, Kaplan AJ, Black J, et al. Changes in heart rate variability, quality of life, and activity in cardiac resynchronization therapy patients: results of the HF-HRV registry. Pacing Clin Electrophysiol 2007;30:56–64.

16. Singh JP, Rosenthal LS, Hranitzky PM, et al. Device diagnostics and long-term clinical outcome in patients receiving cardiac resynchronization therapy. Europace 2009;11:1647–53.

17. Cashion AK, Holmes SL, Arheart KL, et al. Heart rate variability and mortality in patients with end stage renal disease. Nephrol Nurs J 2005;32:173–84.

18. Javorka M, Javorkova J, Tonhajzerova I, et al. Parasympathetic versus sympathetic control of the cardiovascular system in young patients with type 1 diabetes mellitus. Clin Physiol Funct Imaging 2005;25:270–4.

19. Melenovsky V, Simek J, Sperl M, et al. Relation between actual heart rate and autonomic effects of beta blockade in healthy men. Am J Cardiol 2005;95:999–1002.

20. Barutcu I, Esen AM, Kaya D, et al. Cigarette smoking and heart rate variability: dynamic influence of parasympathetic and sympathetic maneuvers. Ann Noninvasive Electrocardiol 2005;10:324–9.

21. Becher J, Kaufmann SG, Paule S, et al. Device-based impedance measurement is a useful and accurate tool for direct assessment of intrathoracic fluid accumulation in heart failure. Europace 2010;12:731–40.

22. Wang L, Lahtinen S, Lentz L, et al. Feasibility of using an implantable system to measure thoracic congestion in an ambulatory chronic heart failure canine model. Pacing Clin Electrophysiol 2005;28:404–11.

23. Yu CM, Wang L, Chau E, et al. Intrathoracic impedance monitoring in patients with heart failure: correlation with fluid status and feasibility of early warning preceding hospitalization. Circulation 2005;112:841–8.

24. Ypenburg C, Bax JJ, van der Wall EE, et al. Intrathoracic impedance monitoring to predict decompensated heart failure. Am J Cardiol 2007;99:554–7.

25. Maines M, Catanzariti D, Cemin C, et al. Usefulness of intrathoracic fluids accumulation monitoring with an implantable biventricular defibrillator in reducing hospitalizations in patients with heart failure: a case-control study. J Interv Card Electrophysiol 2007;19:201–7.

26. Jhanjee R, Templeton GA, Sattiraju S, et al. Relationship of paroxysmal atrial tachyarrhythmias to volume overload: assessment by implanted transpulmonary impedance monitoring. Circ Arrhythm Electrophysiol 2009;2:488–94.

27. Moore HJ, Peters MN, Franz MR, et al. Intrathoracic impedance preceding ventricular tachyarrhythmia episodes. Pacing Clin Electrophysiol 2010;33:960–6.

28. Ip JE, Cheung JW, Park D, et al. Temporal associations between thoracic volume overload and malignant ventricular arrhythmias: a study of intrathoracic impedance. J Cardiovasc Electrophysiol 2011;22:293–9.

29. Maines M, Landolina M, Lunati M, et al, Italian Clinical Service Optivol-CRT Group. Intrathoracic and ventricular impedances are associated with changes in ventricular volume in patients receiving defibrillators for CRT. Pacing Clin Electrophysiol 2010;33:64–73.

30. Whellan DJ, Droogan CJ, Fitzpatrick J, et al. Change in intrathoracic impedance measures during acute decompensated heart failure admission: results from the Diagnostic Data for Discharge in Heart Failure Patients (3D-HF) Pilot Study. J Card Fail 2012;18:107–12.

31. Wang L. Fundamentals of intrathoracic impedance monitoring in heart failure. Am J Cardiol 2007;99:3G–10G.

32. Kramer DB, Maisel WH. An unusual cause of abnormal intrathoracic impedance in a patient with arrhythmogenic right ventricular cardiomyopathy. Pacing Clin Electrophysiol 2011;34:e60–3.

33. van Veldhuisen DJ, Braunschweig F, Conraads V, et al, DOT-HF Investigators. Intrathoracic impedance monitoring, audible patient alerts, and outcome in patients with heart failure. Circulation 2011;124:1719–27.

34. Brachmann J, Böhm M, Rybak K, et al, Study Executive Board and Investigators. Fluid status monitoring with a wireless network to reduce cardiovascular-related hospitalizations and mortality in heart failure: rationale and design of the OptiLink HF Study (Optimization of Heart Failure Management using OptiVol Fluid Status Monitoring and CareLink). Eur J Heart Fail 2011;13:796–804.

35. Zile MR, Bennett TD, St John Sutton M, et al. Transition from chronic compensated to acute decompensated heart failure: pathophysiological insights obtained from continuous monitoring of intracardiac pressures. Circulation 2008;118:1433–41.

36. Troughton R, Ritzema J, Eigle NL, et al. Direct left atrial pressure monitoring in severe heart failure: long-term sensor performance. J Cardiovasc Transl Res 2011;4:3–13.

37. Zehender M, Faber T, Grom A, et al. Continuous monitoring of acute myocardial ischaemia by the implantable cardioverter defibrillator. Am Heart J 1994;127:1057–63.

38. Stadler RW, Lu SN, Nelson SD, et al. A real-time ST-segment monitoring algorithm for implantable devices. J Electrocardiol 2001;34:119–26.

39. Theres H, Stadler RW, Stylos L, et al. Comparison of electrocardiogram and intra-thoracic electrogram signals for detection of ischaemic segment changes during normal sinus and ventricular paced rhythms. J Cardiovasc Electrophysiol 2002;13:990–5.

40. Fischell TA, Fischell DR, Fischell RE, et al. Real-time detection and alerting for acute ST-segment elevation myocardial ischemia using an implantable, high-fidelity, intracardiac electrogram monitoring system with long-range telemetry in an ambulatory porcine model. J Am Coll Cardiol 2006;48:2306–14.

41. Asbach S, Weiss I, Wenzel B, et al. Intrathoracic far-field electrocardiogram allows continuous monitoring of ischemia after total coronary occlusion. Pacing Clin Electrophysiol 2006;29:1334–40.

42. Baron TW, Faber TS, Grom A, et al. Real-time assessment of acute myocardial ischaemia by an intra-thoracic 6-lead ECG: evaluation of a new diagnostic option in the implantable defibrillator. Europace 2006;8:994–1001.

43. Forleo GB, Tesauro M, Panattoni G, et al. Impact of continuous intracardiac ST-segment monitoring on mid-term outcomes of ICD-implanted patients with coronary artery disease. Early results of a prospective comparison with conventional ICD outcomes. Heart 2012;98:402–7.

Leadless Pacing and Defibrillation Systems

Joseph J. Gard, MD, Yong-Mei Cha, MD,
Paul A. Friedman, MD*

KEYWORDS

- Pacemaker • Defibrillator • Leadless • Bradycardia • Tachycardia

KEY POINTS

- With the expanded use cardiac implantable electronic devices, lead-related complications, including electrical malfunction, valvular injury, infectious risks, thrombus formation, and venous stenosis, have become important concerns.
- A totally self-contained intracardiac pacemaker will be available for demand ventricular pacing in the near future, but questions related to battery depletion, dislodgment, magnetic resonance imaging, and coagulum formation remain unanswered.
- Devices that harvest energy from cardiac motion will probably become a reality, although these efforts remain early in their development.
- Technology to permit extracardiac energy delivery to a transducer in the heart has also been demonstrated and may eliminate the need for leads.
- Implantation of biologic tissue to provide pacing support has been demonstrated in large animal models, although many challenges remain.
- The next generation of pacemakers and defibrillators will likely eliminate the current systems' weakest link: the transvenous electrode.

INTRODUCTION

The hazards associated with bradycardia have been known to mankind for more than 2500 years, after Pien Ch'iao in ancient China astutely observed that decreased heartbeats led to an increased risk of death.[1] In the 1800s, Adams[2] and Stokes[3] described syncope in association with bradycardia caused by complete heart block. However, effective therapy was not introduced until the late 1900s, when cardiac pacing was developed and subsequently rapidly adopted in clinical practice.[4] The first pacemaker was implanted in 1958 in a patient who received 26 pulse generators during his life, outliving the surgeon who first inserted his device. Initial systems used surgically placed epicardial leads. The introduction of transvenous leads significantly reduced implant morbidity. Despite remarkable technologic advances since then, modern pacing systems continue to have important limitations, predominantly related to intravascular leads. Leads must survive in the harsh environment of the body, with repeated mechanical stress caused by the beating heart, and potentially deforming bends as they course through the venous system. Leads introduce a large intravascular surface area available for infection and thrombus formation. Leads are at risk for fracture,[5] infection,[6] dislodgement,[7] and functional failure.[8] Leads can also disrupt neighboring anatomy, causing venous stenosis,[9] venous occlusion,[10] and valvular incompetence.[11] Lead extraction to eradicate systemic or device pocket infection, remove nonfunctional or harmful leads,

Relevant Disclosures: None.
Division of Cardiovascular Diseases, Mayo Clinic, 200 First Street Southwest, Rochester, MN 55905, USA
* Corresponding author.
E-mail address: friedman.paul@mayo.edu

Card Electrophysiol Clin 5 (2013) 327–335
http://dx.doi.org/10.1016/j.ccep.2013.05.009

or restore venous flow in the setting of obstruction exposes patients to a substantial risk of morbidity and mortality.[12–14] Leads are considered the weakest link in pacing systems, highlighted by a long history of manufacturer recalls and advisories, with a potentially adverse influence on patients and society. Thus, efforts are ongoing to develop a leadless method for cardiac pacing.

Although efforts to design a leadless pacing system have been longstanding, no system is currently available in clinical practice. Several strategies have evolved over years to eliminate leads, or intracardiac leads, and these are reviewed herein.

THE CONCEPT OF A LEADLESS PACEMAKER

A pacing system must deliver a stimulus to capture the myocardium. The leads in the traditional system function to deliver energy from the pulse generator to the myocardium. To avoid intravascular leads, either the energy must be totally contained in the element placed in the heart (eg, a totally self-contained intracardiac pacemaker[15]) or the energy must be transmitted without an intravascular lead to the stimulation site.

The concept of a totally self-contained intracardiac pacemaker was described in 1970.[15] A nuclear battery allowed the pulse generator to be miniaturized to a size (8 × 18 mm) that could be implanted within the heart (**Fig. 1**). It was implanted successfully in a canine study with pacing at 100 beats per minute for 66 days without any recognized complications.[15] Although this initial prototype did include barbs to anchor the device within the heart, the potential for embolization is a concern with an intracardiac pacemaker. This possibility is particularly relevant in the current era of invasive cardiology, with potential dislodgement during cardiac procedures performed subsequent to intracardiac pacemaker implantation.

DEVELOPMENT OF A MODERN LEADLESS PACEMAKER

Four decades later, new leadless pacemakers with modern design are on the horizon. Medtronic (Medtronic, Minneapolis, MN, USA) has developed a leadless pacemaker prototype that is in early clinical study in humans (**Fig. 2**). This device has a self-contained generator and is 20 F in diameter and 24 mm in length. The device can be delivered to the right ventricle by a 20 F sheath via femoral vein access. The estimated battery life is 7 to 10 years. It is designed for active fixation, with 4 barbs anchoring the device to the endomyocardium, and is retrievable when needed. Animal studies showed stable low pacing thresholds of 0.6 V per 0.5 ms with 20 weeks of observation when the pacemaker was placed in a sheep's right ventricle.[16] The system includes telemetry to permit communication with an external programmer.

Similarly, the Nanostim (Nanostim, Inc., Sunnyvale, CA, USA) leadless pacemaker has completed preclinical investigation. This device is only 1 cm^3 in volume and weighs 2 g; it is as small as a dime (**Fig. 3**). It has active fixation mechanism at the device tip that can be freely extended into or retracted from the myocardium. The battery life is estimated at 7 years, with 100% pacing at 2.5 V output. The current prototype leadless pacemaker offers single-chamber rate adaptive pacing. A clinical study of this device is underway in Europe (ClinicalTrials.gov identifier: NCT01700244). Leadless single-chamber pacing will likely be available in clinical practice in the next 2 to 3 years.

The theoretical strengths of these systems are that they avoid many of the pitfalls of current conventional pacing systems. Leadless systems allow for endocardial pacing, which is more physiologic than epicardial pacing. Although, the devices are being primarily studied for right ventricular pacing,

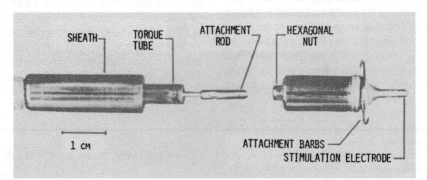

Fig. 1. An early design of a totally self-contained cardiac pacing system. (*From* Spickler W, Rasor NS, Kezdi P, et al. Totally self-contained intracardiac pacemaker. J Electrocardiol 1970;3:325; with permission.)

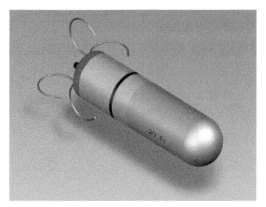

Fig. 2. Modern design of Medtronic intracardiac pace-maker includes barbs for a secure anchor to minimize the risk of dislodgement. (*From* Cheng A, Teresh-chenko LG. Evolutionary innovations in cardiac pac-ing. J Electrocardiol 2011;44:614; with permission.)

assessment of leadless left ventricular pacing is anticipated. For left ventricular pacing, deployment may be into the pericardial space as an epicardial pacing system because of the risk of potentially catastrophic systemic embolization with endocardial left ventricular placement. Moreover, because of the juxtaposition of the left atrial appendage and the left ventricular epicardium, such a device could provide dual-chamber pacing with left atrial to left ventricular synchronization relatively easily, avoiding the challenge of multiple discrete leadless elements that must intercommunicate to ensure appropriate timing of pacing therapy. Surgical delivery of an epicardial pacing system can be performed using video-assisted thoracoscopy,[17] lower half mini sternotomy,[18] or at the time of cardiac surgery via traditional median sternotomy.[19] Another anticipated approach to be developed will be via percutaneous epicardial

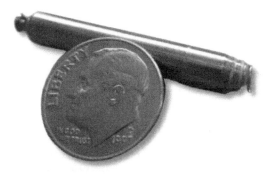

Fig. 3. The small size of the Nanostim leadless intra-cardiac pacemaker is demonstrated with a dime for size reference. (*Courtesy of* Nanostim, Inc, Sunnyvale, CA; with permission.)

access, which invasive electrophysiologists are increasingly using for other electrophysiology procedures, such as epicardial ablation[20] and left atrial appendage closures.

Traditionally, the drawbacks of epicardial leads are the need for surgical placement and the relatively high failure rate over time because of capture threshold elevation.[19] Intramyocardial electrode placement has shown promising results and may avoid this limitation.[21,22] Additionally, percutaneous strategies must avoid inadvertent coronary artery injury.

Leadless pacing strategies face several challenges. One is the inability to provide atrioventricular pacing with a single device (unless placed epicardially). Coordinated atrioventricular pacing will require communication between independently implanted systems using wireless technology, with a potentially significant expense to the battery. Similarly, a system to optimize biventricular function would require communication between a right ventricular device and a left ventricular device. Pulse generator battery depletion is another potential limitation, because removal of a chronically implanted system will likely be very difficult due to endothelialization of the device. Although multiple devices might be placed within a cardiac chamber, the total number may be limited. Whether the moving mass of one or more leadless pulse generators may provoke arrhythmias is unknown, although this has not been reported in early experience. The potential limitations of power have sparked interest in harvesting biologic energy and external power sources.

Harvesting Biologic Energy

One potential source of energy to power pacing system is cardiac motion. This is conceptually very appealing. The pacemaker ultimately receives its power from the meals a person ingests, which in turn are metabolized to provide mechanical energy. Converting mechanical energy to electrical energy is well-known in other disciplines, with common examples including hydroelectric dams and wind electricity. Various basic concepts have been proposed to harness kinetic energy within the cardiovascular system to power a cardiac pacing system. Piezoelectric systems convert the vibrations of heartbeats into electrical energy, which can be used to power pacemakers.[23] Ventricular wall motion can be harnessed by a variable-capacitance–type electrostatic generator, and this concept has been demonstrated in an animal experiment.[24] Another concept is to use pressure responsive bladders to harness the energy from changing cardiac pressures (right atrial and right ventricular pressures) to power a pacing system.[25] All of these approaches are challenged by the limitations in energy yield using current technology. Epicardial systems may have an advantage because of the greater radius of curvature, which may increase the energy extracted. However, the challenges of harvesting cardiac motion and pressure to power electronic systems have sparked interest in external energy sources to power passive elements to transduce energy into pacing stimuli.

REMOTE ENERGY DELIVERY: ULTRASOUND-POWERED PACEMAKER

An alternative to the concept of the totally self-contained intracardiac pacemaker is a system that delivers power wirelessly to an intracardiac component using the body as the medium for power delivery. This concept has been demonstrating using ultrasound energy.[26] An external ultrasound generator was used to transcutaneously deliver energy to a transducer positioned in the heart (**Fig. 4**). The transducer converted the ultrasound energy to

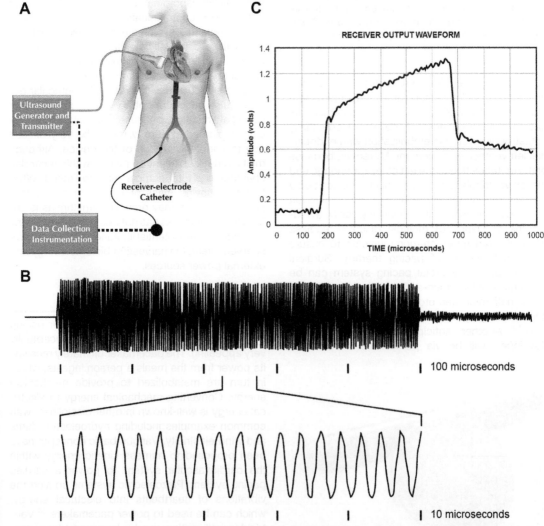

Fig. 4. Delivery of energy from outside of the body through ultrasound transmission to an intracardiac receiver for pacing (*A*). The energy is delivered from the ultrasound generator and transducer by pulses (0.5 ms duration) at a frequency of 350 ± 25 kHz (*B*). The pulse available at the intracardiac catheter is shown (*C*). (*From* Lee KL, Lau CP, Tse HF, et al. First human demonstration of cardiac stimulation with transcutaneous ultrasound energy delivery: implications for wireless pacing with implantable devices. J Am Coll Cardiol 2007;50:877–83; with permission.)

electrical energy used to stimulate the heart. In a feasibility study that enrolled 24 patients at the time of clinical electrophysiologic study, a receiver was mounted on a catheter that was maneuvered to the heart via the femoral vein, and stimulated via external ultrasound at frequencies ranging from 313 to 385 kHz. The ultrasound transmission amplitude was limited to maintain a mechanical index less than 1.9, the maximum permitted for imaging systems. Pacing sites tested included the right atrium, right ventricle, and left ventricle (predominantly endocardial). The mean distance from transmitter to pacing site was 11 cm, the mean mechanical index during pacing was 0.5, and the mean ultrasound mediated capture threshold was 1 V. No adverse events occurred, and no patient discomfort was experienced during pacing. Although not truly leadless because the pacing element was mounted on a catheter, proof of concept was demonstrated, because the transducer component could potentially be implanted in the heart to permit leadless pacing.

A potential limitation of using ultrasound energy may be the lack of a reliable acoustic window for energy transmission, depending on transducer and transmitter locations. Lung fields do not transmit ultrasound, and thus limit the acoustic windows available for transmission to the heart. Furthermore, the acoustic windows may change with body position and respiration. A follow-up study assessed the acoustic window for left ventricular pacing in 10 patients and found it to be adequate in all, permitting acutely successful temporary pacing of the left ventricle via transcutaneously transmitted ultrasound.[27]

BIOLOGIC PACEMAKER

An alternative approach to implanting electronic hardware for leadless pacing is to implant biologically active material to introduce spontaneous electrical discharge in regions of myocardium that would otherwise remain excitable but inactive. In theory, this system could grow and develop with young patients, respond to modulations in autonomic tone, and never require battery replacement. Although proof of concept experiments have been successfully performed in animal models, significant challenges remain, and whether biologic pacemakers will ever supplant electronic devices is unclear.

Biologic pacemakers have been proposed for use in various scenarios: (1) as temporary pacemakers, longer-term cell migration or dysfunction is not a limitation and foreign nonbiologic material is not necessary, which may be advantageous in infections; (2) as hybrid systems, with a biologic pacemaker placed in tandem with an electronic one to provide backup, and the biologic pacemaker providing autonomic responsiveness and mitigating battery depletion; and (3) as replacements to be used instead of electronic pacemakers.[24]

Two broad strategies are used to introduce spontaneous depolarization to regions of otherwise inactive myocardium. Gene therapy involves introducing novel DNA into myocytes, typically using an adenovirus vector to modify ionic currents and generate spontaneous electrical activity.[28] Gene therapy was first studied to treat bradycardia using β_2-adrenergic receptor cDNA.[28] Gene therapy has also been used to modify and balance cellular membrane ion channels.[29] Gene therapy was recently shown to provide effective pacing for 14 days in a porcine model of atrioventricular block.[30] This was achieved through altering the balance of inward rectifier current (I_{K1}) and pacemaker current (I_f).[30]

The genes can be injected into the region of interest, such as the region of the sinus node or atrioventricular node, via a percutaneous approach with a catheter that incorporates a needle delivery system.[31] Stable pacing will likely require modification of various counteracting currents in a carefully controlled manner.[24]

Cell therapy introduces modified mesenchymal stem cells as delivery systems or cells derived from pluripotent stem cells that are created to have sinus node–like function. Use of autologous cells eliminates the need for immunosuppression. Depending on which genes are delivered or cells introduced, the biologic pacemaker may be responsive to the body's neurohumoral mechanisms for heart rate modulation. For example HCN (hyperpolarization-activated, cyclic nucleotide–gated) cation channels are responsive to cyclic adenosine monophosphate, so that altering their expression can develop autonomically responsive pacing (**Fig. 5**).[31]

Although biologic pacemakers are the subject of intense investigation, important challenges remain to their introduction to the clinic. A sufficient number of myocytes must be infected or a large enough number of cells introduced to provide stable pacing. Moreover, gap junctions must form between the stimulating cells and the neighboring myocytes to ensure action potential propagation. Injection site inflammation, cell migration, inadequate rates of transfection, cell migration, and lack of adequate coupling form barriers to effective therapy delivery. Newly injected cells may be rejected or become malignant. The extent of current modification must be carefully titrated; excessive effect may result in dangerous tachycardias, whereas

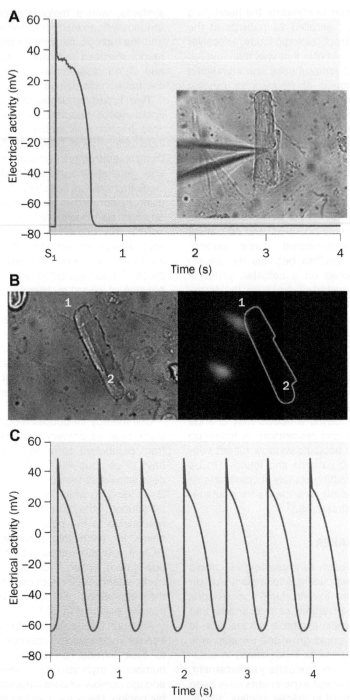

Fig. 5. (*A*) Stimulation of cultured myocytes and HeLa cells that have not been genetically modified results in a single action potential. (*B*) The cultured cells include both myocytes and HeLa cells transfected to expressive connexin 43, green fluorescence protein (GFP), and hyperpolarization-activated, cyclic nucleotide–gated potassium channel 2 (HCN2). (*C*) After genetic modification of connexin 43, GFP, and HCN2, the cells express spontaneous automaticity. (*From* Rosen MR, Robinson RB, Brink PR, et al. The road to biologic pacing. Nat Rev Cardiol 2011;8:659; with permission.)

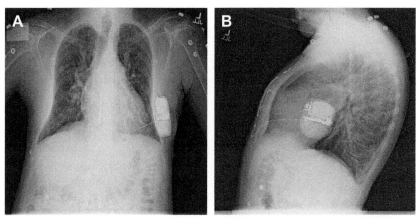

Fig. 6. Chest radiograph showing a subcutaneous defibrillator system in posteroanterior (PA) (*A*) and lateral (*B*) projection. The shocking coil lies parallel to and along the left border of the sternum, with the generator near the apex of the heart inferior to the axilla.

insufficient modification may lead to persistent bradycardia. Although biologic pacemakers remain a hope for the future, significant hurdles remain.

Subcutaneous Implantable Cardioverter Defibrillator

The risk of transvenous lead failure in implantable cardioverter defibrillators (ICDs) exceeds that of pacemaker lead failure.[32] In 2012, the US Food and Drug Administration approved a subcutaneous ICD (S-ICD) that lacks an intravascular component. This system is composed of a generator implanted near the left midaxillary line and a single subcutaneous lead that is tunneled to the midsternum (**Fig. 6**). Two electrodes on the lead and the can itself are used to provide 3 possible sensing vectors, and novel detection algorithms discriminate supraventricular tachycardia from ventricular tachycardia. The major advantages of this system stem from the absence of an intravascular lead, potentially limiting morbidity and mortality related to device infections, avoiding the risk for venous occlusion, eliminating injury to the tricuspid valve, obviating the risk of cardiac perforation, and permitting defibrillation therapy in patients with

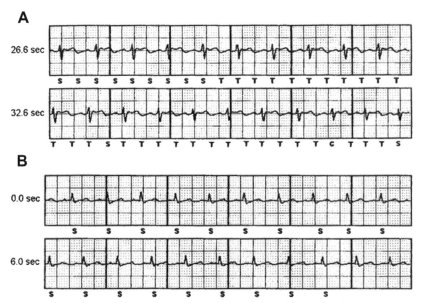

Fig. 7. Inappropriate and appropriate sensing by a subcutaneous defibrillator. (*A*) T-wave oversensing leads to a patient experiencing an inappropriate shock. Changing the sensing vector setting from the secondary sensing vector to the primary sensing vector led to appropriate sensing (*B*).

right to left intracardiac shunts without introducing a risk of stroke.

The S-ICD is capable of detecting and terminating life-threatening ventricular tachycardia and fibrillation with shocks of up to 80 J. A limitation of this system, however, is the lack of bradycardia and antitachycardia pacing capability. Although the system is not designed for bradycardic support, it does provide 30 seconds of cardiac pacing after a shock triggered by a 3.5-second pause. Thus, the S-ICD is a reasonable therapeutic consideration in patients who meet conventional ICD indications and do not have an indication for cardiac pacing or resynchronization.

Bardy and colleagues[33] reported favorable early experience with the S-ICD. Defibrillation thresholds are typically higher with the S-ICD than with transvenous systems, because of the greater distance between defibrillation electrodes and myocardium, resulting in the need for a larger pulse generator.[33] Although small, nonrandomized studies have suggested similar efficacy and complication rates with the S-ICD and transvenous ICDs,[34,35] but prospective randomized trials are lacking.[36] Early experience is promising, but troubleshooting and system optimization is occasionally required (**Fig. 7**).

SUMMARY

Cardiac implantable electronic devices have evolved from simple ventricular pacing to prevent Stokes-Adams attacks from high-grade atrioventricular block to sophisticated systems capable of treating bradycardias, heart failure, syncope, and tachyarrhythmias. With their expanded use, lead-related complications, including electrical malfunction, valvular injury, infectious risks, thrombus formation, and venous stenosis, have become important concerns. Emerging novel systems may mitigate or eliminate these complications. Totally self-contained intracardiac pacemakers will be available for demand ventricular pacing in the near future, but questions related to battery depletion, dislodgment, magnetic resonance imaging, and coagulum formation remain unanswered. Devices that harvest energy from cardiac motion will likely become a reality, although efforts remain early in development. Technology to permit extracardiac energy delivery to a transducer in the heart has also been demonstrated, and may eliminate the need for leads. Implantation of biologic tissue to provide pacing support has been shown in large animal models, although many challenges remain. The next generation of pacemakers and defibrillators will likely eliminate the current systems' weakest link: the transvenous electrode.

REFERENCES

1. Scherf D, Schott A. Extrasystoles and allied arrhythmias. Chicago: Year Book Medical Publishers; 1973.
2. Adams R. Cases of diseases of the heart accompanied with pathological observations. Dublin Hospital Reports 1827;4:353–453.
3. Stokes W. Observations on some cases of permanently slow pulse. Dublin Quarterly Journal of Medical Science 1846;2:73–85.
4. Gregoratos G, Abrams J, Epstein AE, et al. ACC/AHA/NASPE 2002 guideline update for implantation of cardiac pacemakers and antiarrhythmia devices: summary article. Circulation 2002;106(16): 2145–61.
5. Alt E, Volker R, Blomer H. Lead fracture in pacemaker patients. Thorac Cardiovasc Surg 1987; 35(2):101–4.
6. Lo R, D'Anca M, Cohen T, et al. Incidence and prognosis of pacemaker lead-associated masses: a study of 1,569 transesophageal echocardiograms. J Invasive Cardiol 2006;18(12):599–601.
7. Cheng A, Wang Y, Curtis JP, et al. Acute lead dislodgements and in-hospital mortality in patients enrolled in the national cardiovascular data registry implantable cardioverter defibrillator registry. J Am Coll Cardiol 2010;56(20):1651–6.
8. Birnie DH, Parkash R, Exner DV, et al. Clinical predictors of fidelis lead failure: a report from the Canadian Heart Rhythm Society Device Committee. Circulation 2012;125(10):1217–25.
9. Rozmus G, Daubert JP, Huang DT, et al. Venous thrombosis and stenosis after implantation of pacemakers and defibrillators. J Interv Card Electrophysiol 2005;13(1):9–19.
10. Riezebos RK, Schroeder-Tanka J, de Voogt WG. Occlusion of the proximal subclavian vein complicating pacemaker lead implantation. Europace 2006;8(1):42–3.
11. Lin G, Nishimura RA, Connolly HM, et al. Severe symptomatic tricuspid valve regurgitation due to permanent pacemaker or implantable cardioverter-defibrillator leads. J Am Coll Cardiol 2005;45(10): 1672–5.
12. Maytin M, Jones SO, Epstein LM. Long-term mortality after transvenous lead extraction. Circ Arrhythm Electrophysiol 2012;5(2):252–7.
13. Jones SO 4th, Eckart RE, Albert CM, et al. Large, single-center, single-operator experience with transvenous lead extraction: outcomes and changing indications. Heart Rhythm 2008;5(4):520–5.
14. Bongiorni MG, Soldati E, Zucchelli G, et al. Transvenous removal of pacing and implantable cardiac defibrillating leads using single sheath mechanical dilatation and multiple venous approaches: high success rate and safety in more than 2000 leads. Eur Heart J 2008;29(23):2886–93.

15. Spickler JW, Rasor NS, Kezdi P, et al. Totally self-contained intracardiac pacemaker. J Electrocardiol 1970;3(3–4):325–31.

16. Bonner MD, Eggen MD. Chronic animal study of leadless pacer design. Heart Rhythm 2011;8(5):S1.

17. Nelson KE, Bates MG, Turley AJ, et al. Video-assisted thoracoscopic left ventricular pacing in patients with and without previous sternotomy. Ann Thorac Surg 2013;95(3):907–13.

18. Hosseini MT, Popov AF, Kourliouros A, et al. Surgical implantation of a biventricular pacing system via lower half mini sternotomy. J Cardiothorac Surg 2013;8:5.

19. Helguera ME, Maloney JD, Woscoboinik JR, et al. Long-term performance of epimyocardial pacing leads in adults: comparison with endocardial leads. Pacing Clin Electrophysiol 1993;16(3 Pt 1):412–7.

20. d'Avila A, Koruth JS, Dukkipati S, et al. Epicardial access for the treatment of cardiac arrhythmias. Europace 2012;14(Suppl 2):ii13–8.

21. Asirvatham SJ, Bruce CJ, Danielsen A, et al. Intra-myocardial pacing and sensing for the enhancement of cardiac stimulation and sensing specificity. Pacing Clin Electrophysiol 2007;30(6):748–54.

22. Henz BD, Friedman PA, Bruce CJ, et al. Synchronous ventricular pacing without crossing the tricuspid valve or entering the coronary sinus–preliminary results. J Cardiovasc Electrophysiol 2009; 20(12):1391–7.

23. Karami MA, Inman DJ. Powering pacemakers from heartbeat vibrations using linear and nonlinear energy harvesters. Appl Phys Lett 2012;100:042901.

24. Tashiro R, Kabei N, Katayama K, et al. Development of an electrostatic generator for a cardiac pacemaker that harnesses the ventricular wall motion. J Artif Organs 2002;5:239–45.

25. Roberts P, Stanley G, Morgan JM. Abstract 2165: harvesting the energy of cardiac motion to power a pacemaker. Circulation 2008;118:S679–80.

26. Lee KL, Lau CP, Tse HF, et al. First human demonstration of cardiac stimulation with transcutaneous ultrasound energy delivery: implications for wireless pacing with implantable devices. J Am Coll Cardiol 2007;50(9):877–83.

27. Lee KL, Tse HF, Echt DS, et al. Temporary leadless pacing in heart failure patients with ultrasound-mediated stimulation energy and effects on the acoustic window. Heart Rhythm 2009;6(6):742–8.

28. Rajesh G, Francis J. Biological pacemakers. Indian Pacing Electrophysiol J 2006;6(1):1–5.

29. Rosen MR, Brink PR, Cohen IS, et al. The road to biological pacing. Nat Rev Cardiol 2011;8(11): 656–66.

30. Cingolani E, Yee K, Shehata M, et al. Biological pacemaker created by percutaneous gene delivery via venous catheters in a porcine model of complete heart block. Heart Rhythm 2012;9(8):1310–8.

31. Cho HC, Marban E. Biological therapies for cardiac arrhythmias: can genes and cells replace drugs and devices? Circ Res 2010;106(4):674–85.

32. Maisel WH, Kramer DB. Implantable cardioverter-defibrillator lead performance. Circulation 2008; 117:2721–3.

33. Bardy GH, Smith WM, Hood MA, et al. An entirely subcutaneous implantable cardioverter-defibrillator. N Engl J Med 2010;363(1):36–44.

34. Olde Nordkamp LR, Dabiri Abkenari L, Boersma LV, et al. The entirely subcutaneous implantable cardioverter-defibrillator: initial clinical experience in a large Dutch cohort. J Am Coll Cardiol 2012; 60(19):1933–9.

35. Kobe J, Reinke F, Meyer C, et al. Implantation and follow-up of totally subcutaneous versus conventional implantable cardioverter-defibrillators: a multicenter case-control study. Heart Rhythm 2013;10(1):29–36.

36. Hauser RG. The subcutaneous implantable cardioverter-defibrillator: should patients want one? J Am Coll Cardiol 2013;61(1):20–2.

Remote Device Management in Patients with Cardiac Complaints

Haran Burri, MD[a], Niraj Varma, MA, DM, FRCP[b],*

KEYWORDS

- Remote monitoring • Pacemaker • Implantable cardioverter-defibrillator
- Implantable loop recorder • Cardiac symptoms

KEY POINTS

- Remote monitoring systems differ (patient activated vs automatic).
- Automatic remote monitoring maintains constant surveillance, enabling same-day alerts of problems that may underlie cardiac symptoms.
- Remote monitoring prevents unnecessary hospital visits; these are reserved only for those patients who require this. This ability is useful to patients and increases clinic efficiencies.
- Many different sensors are under development (eg, for ischemia and heart failure).

INTRODUCTION

Cardiac implantable electronic devices (CIEDs) treat bradyarrhythmias, and tachyarrhythmias, and heart failure but also record a wealth of data that may be used to help manage patients. These data may be consulted during in-office follow-up or remotely via Web-based platforms. Remote CIED management includes remote follow-up (which involves scheduled automatic device interrogations), remote monitoring (which involves automatic unscheduled transmission of alerts; eg, for atrial fibrillation [AF]), and patient-initiated interrogations (which are full device interrogations initiated manually by the patient; eg, in response to symptoms). All three functions are important for handling patients with cardiac complaints. Furthermore, external databases generated by remote monitoring systems are not subject to saturation or overwritten memory counters within the implantable device, improving accuracy of gathered data and enabling improvement in diagnostic yield. An understanding of all these modes of operation, and functional differences among proprietary platforms, is essential for correct application to those patients with cardiac complaints.

TECHNOLOGIES

Modern implantable cardioverter-defibrillators (ICDs) and some pacemakers (PMs) from major device companies have wireless capabilities that allow them to automatically communicate with a transmitter unit installed at the patient's home, which then relays the data to a secure database (**Fig. 1**). The data are available for consultation by

Disclosures: H.B. receives research grants, fellowship support, and speaker honoraria from Biotronik, Boston Scientific, Medtronic, St-Jude Medical, and Sorin, and was funded in part by a grant from the La Tour Foundation for Cardiovascular Research. N.V. receives research grants, fellowship support, and speaker honoraria from Biotronik, Boston Scientific, Medtronic, and St-Jude Medical.

[a] Electrophysiology Unit, University Hospital of Geneva, Rue Perret-Gentil 4, Geneva 14, CH 1211, Switzerland;
[b] Cardiac Pacing and Electrophysiology, Heart and Vascular Institute, Cleveland Clinic, 9500 Euclid Avenue, Cleveland, OH 44195, USA
* Corresponding author.
E-mail address: varman@ccf.org

Card Electrophysiol Clin 5 (2013) 337–347
http://dx.doi.org/10.1016/j.ccep.2013.05.005
1877-9182/13/$ – see front matter © 2013 Elsevier Inc. All rights reserved.

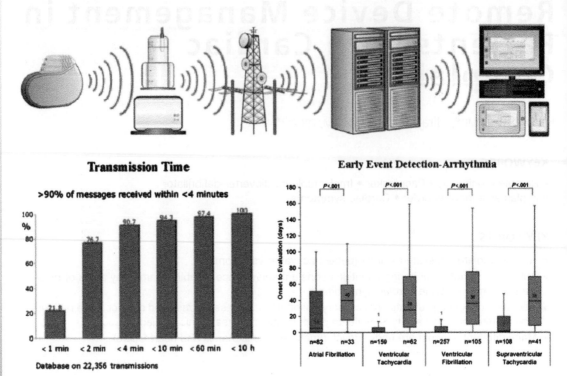

Fig. 1. Automatic remote monitoring technology. (*Top*) Transmission steps in this fully automatic system. Very-low-power radiofrequency transmitter circuitry integrated within the pulse generator wirelessly transmits stored data on a daily basis to a mobile communicator (typically placed bedside at night). The data are relayed wirelessly or via landline (automatically seeking the first path available) to a service center. The wireless transmission ability is especially useful because currently almost 20% (and increasing) of US households are estimated to have no landline facility. The service center receives incoming data and automatically generates a customized summary, available to the physician online via secure Internet access. Critical event data may be transmitted immediately and flagged for attention on the Web page. (*Bottom left*) With home monitoring, more than 90% of transmissions were received in less than 5 minutes with 100% preservation of data integrity. (*Bottom right*) Time to physician evaluation of arrhythmias in the TRUST trial. This technology provides the ability for early detection and enables prompt clinical intervention, if necessary. (*Adapted from* Refs.[4,5,32]; with permission.)

the physician, who can therefore remotely manage the patient and the device. The different systems function in a similar manner, although they have technical differences. Older implantable devices require a telemetry wand for manual interrogation by the patient, which is a setback, especially for children and the elderly.[1] Recent implantable devices have an incorporated antenna that allows wireless automatic data transmission with a unit installed in the patient's home. The requirement for patient participation is minimal for most systems (and, in some, none except for correctly installing the system). The data are sent via landline phone or the GSM (Global System for Mobile Communications) network to a secure database server. A message is then sent to the physician by e-mail, SMS (Short Message Service), or by fax (depending on the system and its configuration), who may then consult the data via a secured Internet access.

The importance of being cognizant of different remote platforms was shown in a recent report from the Cleveland Clinic describing workflow over a 2-week period. Forty-nine percent of all of scheduled remote transmissions were missed because of patient noncompliance.[2] Most of the patients were equipped with systems that require manual transmission over a landline. Automatic wireless systems may resolve many of these problems, but may differ regarding reliability of data transfer and any requirement for patient interaction. In the CONNECT trial (Clinical evaluation of remote notification to reduce time to clinical decision trial),[3] 45% of the automatic clinician alerts were not successfully transmitted, mainly because the home transmitter was not correctly set up or connected to a phone line. This failure limits the role as an early warning mechanism. In contrast, with another remote monitoring platform in the TRUST trial[4] using a mobile wireless transmitter with a simple and automatic setup process, 91% of the daily transmissions were successfully transmitted to the device clinic, ensuring that recently refreshed data were automatically available for review at any stage. Event notifications with this system were delivered in less than 4 minutes (see **Fig. 1**).[5,6] These strengths are significant and this proprietary technology was approved specifically for early detection (http://www.fda.gov/Medical Devices/ProductsandMedicalProcedures/Device ApprovalsandClearances/PMAApprovals/ucm 166550.htm). In addition to these technical aspects, patient education in implementing remote device management will also affect adoption of the technology. None of the existing systems currently allow remote programming of the implanted device. However, during remote follow-up, patients may receive notification via the receiver (callback function, third-party arrhythmia service, or live interaction), which may be reassuring.

There is solid evidence that remote device follow-up can safely supplant a large proportion of routine in-office visits, which are burdensome to patients and pose significant barriers to sustained surveillance.[3,4,7] The TRUST trial showed that transferring from a conventional protocol of only in-person follow-up to a system of remote follow-up with only yearly scheduled in-person evaluations reduced the volume of hospital interactions by almost 50%. Adherence to continued follow-up improved with the remote system, likely because of greater convenience. At the same time, remote monitoring dramatically reduced time to identify clinically significant events. The ability to notify asymptomatic problems that may presage symptomatic device-related or disease-related problems provides a mechanism for preemptive intervention.

REMOTELY MANAGED IMPLANTABLE LOOP RECORDERS: SYNCOPE AND AF

Implantable loop recorders (ILRs) have significant applications to patients for conditions such as unexplained syncope,[8] cryptogenic stroke, palpitations, or for monitoring recurrence of AF following ablation. These are single-lead electrocardiograph (ECG) monitors that are implanted subcutaneously and are capable of storing ECG data on patient activation or automatically, according to predefined bradyarrhythmia or tachyarrhythmia criteria (**Fig. 2**). Their battery longevity is several years. The currently available devices are the Reveal DX/XT (Medtronic, Minneapolis, MN), Confirm DM2100/DM2102 (St-Jude Medical, St Paul, MN), and the Biomonitor (Biotronik, Berlin, Germany; just recently launched in Europe and not yet available in the United States). Both the Reveal and Confirm ILRs are capable of

manual data transmission with a wand via the Care-Link and Merlin.net networks, respectively, whereas the Biomonitor also features automatic wireless transmissions via the Home Monitoring Network. A fourth device, the Sleuth (Transoma Medical, Arden Hills, MN) also has automatic wireless data transmission and received US Food and Drug Administration approval in 2009, but was discontinued the same year when the company closed down for financial reasons.

Despite the apparent appeal of ILRs, their main limitation is suboptimal R-wave detection with either undersensing or oversensing (especially of myopotentials), leading to memory overflow. This limitation adds to the burden of follow-up, and impairs diagnostic yield because clinically significant arrhythmic events may be overwritten. For instance, despite a software upgrade of the Reveal XT, 69% of interrogations had events with artifacts and 32% had storage overflow.[9] Solutions to this problem will be to improve the quality of the signals (which are nevertheless always likely to be hampered by myopotentials), or to transmit data remotely before they are overwritten in the device memory. In a study of 47 patients implanted with a Reveal ILR who were remotely followed up by the CareLink network, weekly manual data transmissions were requested with additional transmissions in case of symptoms.[10] Despite remote data management, ILR storage overflow was observed in 14% of the transmissions. It was nevertheless estimated that, in the absence of CareLink transmissions, saturation of the ILR would have occurred in 45% of patients. Although remote ILR management was positively perceived by the patients in this study, 24% admitted to having sometimes failed to perform transmissions, which underlines the importance of patient compliance, especially in case of nonwireless systems that require manual transmissions with a wand. Automatic wireless transmissions are therefore an important step forward in ensuring maximum diagnostic yield of these devices. This solution may limit data loss caused by memory overflow, but there is still the problem of having to handle large quantities of information. For instance, in a study[9] of 40 patients implanted with the Transoma Sleuth device and followed up for 8.5 ± 5.1 months, a total of 223,226 ECG recordings were transmitted to a monitoring center (an average of 660 per patient per month). Algorithmic filtering eliminated 191,305 (89%) ECGs as artifact. The monitoring center analyzed 31,921 strips and selected 117 (0.37%) ECGs for further evaluation by the physician. This example underlines the importance of improving signal recording and processing by ILRs to alleviate the burden of follow-up.

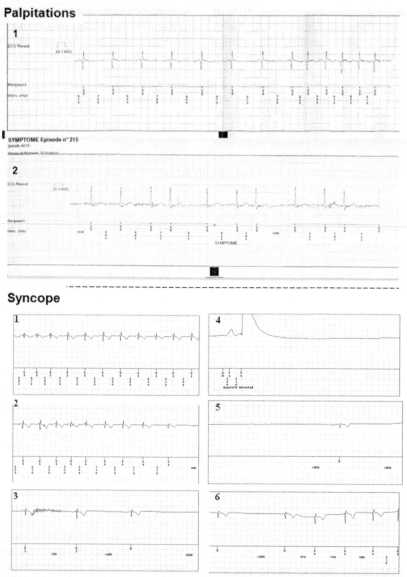

Fig. 2. (*Top*) (*1*) AF onset recorded by a Reveal XT implantable loop recorder in a patient monitored for crypto-genic stroke. (*2*) AF episode in another patient who activated the device because of palpitations. Note the presence of myopotentials on the tracing, which were not sensed in this case. (*Bottom*) (*1–6*) An automatic recording from a Reveal DX catching a 3-second asystole episode in a patient with recurrent falls. The patient passed out and, when she hit the ground, the vector in the episode changed abruptly. She received a pacemaker.

REMOTE MONITORING OF SPECIFIC SYMPTOMS AND CONDITIONS

Syncope

ILRs are playing a growing role in the work-up of patients with syncope and are indicated in patients with recurrent or high-risk syncope of uncertain cause, or to assess the contribution of bradycardia before embarking on cardiac pacing in patients with suspected or certain reflex syncope presenting with frequent or traumatic syncopal episodes.[8,11] There are a multitude of studies on

ILRs in the setting of syncope, with a diagnostic yield ranging from 26%[12] to 94%.[13] However, data are sparse on the remote management of these devices, and no randomized studies exist on how this monitoring strategy may affect diagnostic yield and patient outcome. As mentioned earlier, diagnostic yield is likely to be increased by remote data transmission, because this will reduce the effect of device memory overflow and will also allow earlier detection of programming issues that need to be corrected (especially early after device implantation, when most detection problems are identified). Outcome is also likely to be improved by timely diagnosis of potentially lethal events such as asystole (**Fig. 2**, bottom) or ventricular arrhythmias. In a study with Reveal ILRs, it was estimated that routine weekly manual data transmissions allowed a reduction in time to diagnosis by 71 ± 17 days compared with the usual clinical practice of 3-monthly in-office follow-up.[10] In a study with the Sleuth device (which performs automatic wireless transmissions), data transmission after syncope was within minutes to hours.[14] Other factors, such as responsiveness of the remote monitoring clinic, also determine delay to diagnosis, clinical decisions, and effectiveness.

There are few data on remote monitoring of PMs and ICDs in patients with syncope (**Fig. 3**). In addition to ventricular arrhythmias detected by the device, other causes of syncope such as increase in capture threshold, oversensing, and lead dysfunction may be monitored. In the TRUST trial, delay to evaluation of lead issues was decreased from 23.6 ± 40.2 days in patients with conventional care compared with 4.4 ± 9.2 days on remote monitoring.[15] Same-day discovery occurred in 51%. In a study on 54 patients requiring ICD lead revisions, the 11 patients on remote monitoring had less symptomatic pacing inhibition (eg, caused by T-wave oversensing) compared with the 43 patients without remote surveillance.[16]

Palpitations

Recording of atrial or ventricular arrhythmias is usually performed automatically by CIEDs (as long as they fulfill rate and duration criteria), but correlation with symptoms may be difficult to ascertain. Automatic remote transmission of the events may be useful because they may report events antecedent to symptoms, and thus reduce the delay between symptoms and the event as well as providing valuable diagnostic information. Some PMs allow programming of electrogram recordings during magnet application. Patient-activated remote transmissions may have considerable usefulness here, being useful for rhythm identification during palpitations. However, this requires the patient to have a magnet readily available to capture the event.

In patients without a CIED, Holter monitoring and external loop recorders are the most frequently used diagnostic tools, and ILRs are seldom implanted for this indication.[8]

AF

Remote monitoring of AF has the potential to reduce stroke, inappropriate shocks, and cardiac decompensation. Delay to diagnosis and clinical action probably determines the effect on outcome and has been shown to be dramatically reduced by remote monitoring compared with standard follow-up.[3,4] Potential benefits during modeling suggested that daily monitoring may reduce the 2-year stroke risk by 9% to 18% with an absolute reduction of 0.2% to 0.6% compared with conventional intervisit intervals of 6 to 12 months.[17] In the COMPAS trial,[7] patients on home monitoring had a significantly reduced risk of hospitalization for atrial arrhythmias or stroke ($P<.05$, although COMPAS was not powered to test this hypothesis). Remote monitoring may also offer alternative treatment strategies. The IMPACT trial[18] is currently underway to determine whether on-demand anticoagulation guided by remote monitoring is a safe alternative to continuous anticoagulation.

Monitoring of AF recurrence following ablation has important implications for discontinuing anticoagulation. Perception of AF by patients may change following the procedure, with as many as 37% of patients with recurrences having only asymptomatic episodes.[19] Dual-chamber PMs and ICDs provide full disclosure for AF and are the best method available, especially if remote monitoring is implemented, but do not justify implantation for this purpose per se. Reveal XT ILRs (**Fig. 2**, top panels) have been shown to diagnose AF with 96% sensitivity and 85% specificity compared with simultaneous 48-hour Holter recordings[20] and are currently being evaluated in a trial to remotely monitor patients following AF ablation.[21] The Confirm DM2102 and the Biomonitor ILRs are also capable of diagnosing AF based on RR interval irregularity, but the accuracy of their algorithms has not yet been reported. An issue remains for diagnosing atrial flutter with regular atrioventricular conduction, which may be missed by these devices. In addition, sensing issues such as myopotential oversensing leading to memory overload and increased follow-up burden remains problematic, as discussed earlier.

Dyspnea and Edema

Remote monitoring of heart failure status through parameters such as heart rate, daily activity, and transthoracic impedance has the potential to improve patient outcome. The ability to intervene early with device reprogramming (eg, for loss of biventricular pacing or increased right ventricular pacing) or for arrhythmias (eg, AF) may prevent acute heart failure decompensation (**Fig. 4**). Data analyzed as secondary end points from several trials are encouraging. The CONNECT trial[3]

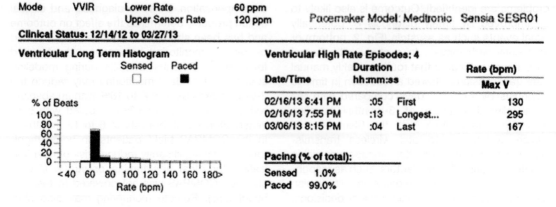

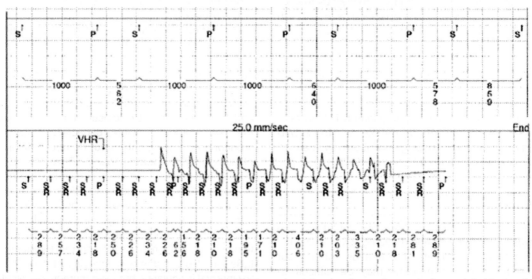

Ventricular High Rate Episode Collected: 02/16/13 7:55 PM

25.0 mm/sec   End

Fig. 3. This 62-year-old woman had a pacemaker implanted previously after atrioventricular nodal ablation for permanent AF. She had had a diarrheal illness for 3 months with weight loss. In February she had episodes of presyncope caused by nonsustained ventricular tachycardia noted in device diagnostics, but only revealed when she scheduled wanded remote follow-up transmission in March, following which she was admitted immediately. A pacemaker with automatic remote monitoring (eg, HM or Merlin) would have initiated an alert notification at time of occurrence. Her potassium on admission was 2.7 mM. HM, home monitoring. (*From* Varma N. Remote monitoring of ICDs and CRTs. Journal of Arrhythmia 2013;29:144–52; with permission.)

randomized 1997 patients implanted with dual-chamber or biventricular ICDs to either remote monitoring or clinic visits, with an 18% reduction ($P = .002$) in the length of cardiovascular hospitalizations in the remote monitoring group. Incorporation of specific hemodynamic sensors may improve preemptive capability. When tested as a standalone unit, a pulmonary artery pressure sensor improved heart failure management (ie, action taken on remotely acquired data benefited patients).[22] Combining different diagnostic parameters (rather than relying on a single parameter) may improve risk stratification of patients.[23] Transferring this computing responsibility from the implanted unit (necessarily limited) to an external service center is an important advantage of wirelessly transmitted data with high frequency. Access to Internet-based information systems provides a framework for multidisciplinary communication and collaboration (eg, with heart failure specialists) and potentially has a critical role in reducing heart failure burden.[24] Analysis of the large ALTITUDE database suggested that patients with heart failure engaged in active remote monitoring networks derived survival advantage.[25]

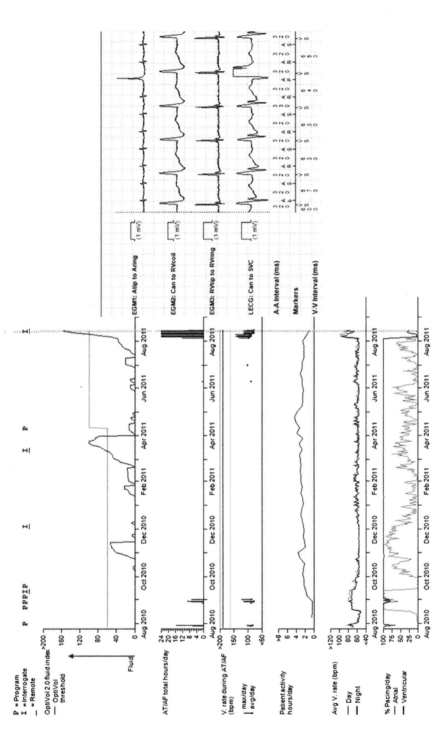

Fig. 4. Remote monitoring alert in a patient with onset of an atrial flutter (visible on the electrogram on the right of the panel) leading to increased heart rates, reduction in ventricular pacing, and an increase in the Optivol lung fluid index (not available in the United States). Note that a previous false-positive Optivol alert (around April 2011) resulted in programming a higher alert threshold.

Chest Pain

Many patients with CIEDs have coronary artery disease, and there has recently been interest to monitor ST segment shifts recorded from unipolar electrograms (right ventricular lead tip to can) for early diagnosis of myocardial ischemia (**Fig. 5**). The AngelMed Guardian implantable ischemia detection system (Angel Medical Systems, Shrewsbury, NJ; currently available only in Brazil) resembles a pacemaker with a standard pacing lead, and monitors beat-to-beat shifts in the ST segment. In case of predefined deviations from average values, vibratory and audible alerts are triggered to prompt the patient to seek medical attention, which may be useful for diagnosis in patients with atypical chest pain (or silent ischemia). The first human experience has been reported in 37 patients over a median follow-up of 1.5 years, of whom 4 patients had ST segment alerts that led to immediate hospital monitoring, with subsequent coronary angiography that confirmed thrombotic coronary occlusion/ruptured plaque.[26] There were 2 false-positive alerts caused by arrhythmias. In a study with 53 patients implanted with a commercially available St-Jude Medical ICD capable of ST segment monitoring, there was no significant clinical benefit in these patients compared with 50 patients implanted with an ICD without this capability, and unscheduled evaluations were increased.[27] The role of remote monitoring in the context of chest pain is questionable, because ST-elevation myocardial infarction requires immediate medical attention, and is best driven by the patient in the interest of time. It may be useful to prevent unnecessary hospital presentation with noncardiac chest pains. However, the sensitivity and specificity of intracardiac ST-elevation for identifying myocardial ischemia require careful determination before executing clinical decisions on this remote alert.

Device Function

Remote monitoring enables potentially same-day discovery of device-related issues.[6] It may facilitate management of unscheduled encounters provoked by device-related symptoms. For example, an appropriate or phantom ICD shock could be managed simply with a reassuring telephone conversation. However, in-person evaluation may be recommended if the physician and/or patient expressed any reservation regarding reconciliation of stated symptoms with remotely acquired data. There is increasing patient concern regarding the function of their implanted devices, despite the great overall reliability of implantable technology in general. Patients who have received inappropriate shocks or who have been informed of recalled components may be particularly apprehensive. In this regard, remote monitoring (rather than remote follow-up at preset intervals) is especially assuring. Notification received during continuous monitoring permits prompt decision making regarding management and, for example, surgical intervention for lead failure (**Fig. 6**), or, conservatively, permits reprogramming to prevent potential inappropriate therapies.[15] In one assessment of lead failure

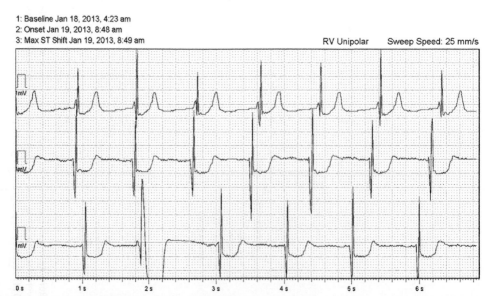

1: Baseline Jan 18, 2013, 4:23 am
2: Onset Jan 19, 2013, 8:48 am
3: Max ST Shift Jan 19, 2013, 8:49 am   RV Unipolar   Sweep Speed: 25 mm/s

Fig. 5. Alert notification received on Merlin.net for ST segment shift in a 57-year-old man with an prophylactic ICD implanted for ischemic cardiomyopathy. (*From* Varma N. Remote monitoring of ICDs and CRTs. Journal of Arrhythmia 2013;29:144–52; with permission.)

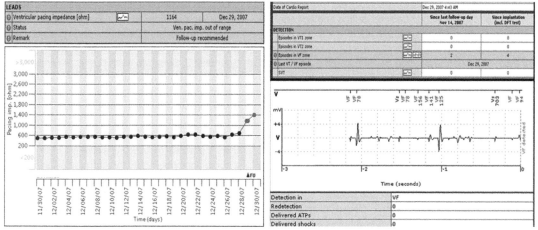

Fig. 6. Home monitoring generator coupled to a lead under class 1 recall (Fidelis, MDT 6949). Two separate event notifications that were transmitted immediately on occurrence of lead fracture, occurring silently during sleep at 4:43 AM, 6 weeks after last clinic follow-up on November 14. (*Left*) Lead impedance suddenly increased; (*Right*) Ventricular fibrillation detection caused by irregular sensed events. Electrogram definition in current generation has improved resolution (1/128 second) and includes postdetection sequences (eg, see **Fig. 2**). The patient was reviewed within hours (FU) of the notifications. This case shows the value of continuous monitoring for rapid identification and correction of recalls and advisories. (*Adapted from* Varma N, Johnson MA. Prevalence of cancelled shock therapy and relationship to shock delivery in recipients of implantable cardioverter-defibrillators assessed by remote monitoring. Pacing Clin Electrophysiol 2009;32(Suppl 1):S42–6; with permission.)

(54 patients), 80% of patients were asymptomatic at the first episode of oversensing, and symptomatic problems were reduced with those managed remotely (27.3%) versus conventionally (53.4%, $P = .04$). Events were notified 54 days after the last ICD interrogation and 56 days before the next scheduled visit (ie, reaction time was advanced by almost 2 months to avoid adverse events). The nonsustained ventricular arrhythmia notification may be triggered by system issues such as lead electrical noise artifacts caused by fracture or nonphysiologic electrical signals, and direct intervention to preempt shock delivery and reduce patient morbidity.[15,28] Interruption of repeated charge cycles, which occur in a significant minority of patients with ICDs,[29] is important to prevent early battery exhaustion. The multicenter ECOST trial confirmed many of these preliminary observations.[30] Clinical reactions enabled by early detection resulted in a large reduction in the number of delivered shocks (−72%), the number of charged shocks (−76%), and the rate of inappropriate shocks (−52%), and at the same time exerted a favorable impact on battery longevity. Reduced generator replacements, aside from cost issues, avoid the considerable morbidity associated with this surgery.[31] Remote care does not supplant the important in-person follow-up in 2 to 12 weeks after implantation, which permits assessment of wound healing, determination of chronic thresholds, and setting of eventual pacing parameters. Lead problems requiring revision and symptomatic reactions

to implantation (eg, pacemaker syndrome, diaphragmatic pacing, and pocket infection) cluster in this early postimplant period and may not be revealed by remote monitoring. However, during subsequent follow-up, current results show considerable superiority of remote monitoring compared with standard follow-up.

SUMMARY

Cardiac ILRs, PMs, and ICDs offer several parameters that may be monitored remotely to manage patients with cardiac complaints, and significantly reduce delay to diagnosis of clinically significant events. This monitoring model has potential usefulness for management of patients with syncope, cryptogenic stroke, AF recurrence after ablation or treatment of heart failure, and for device-related issues. One of the remaining challenges is to ensure that remote monitoring systems are properly set up and used by patients and also that following facilities adopt changes in workflow patterns to efficiently gather and respond to transmitted data without adding to their follow-up burden.

REFERENCES

1. Zartner P, Handke R, Photiadis J, et al. Performance of an autonomous telemonitoring system in children and young adults with congenital heart diseases. Pacing Clin Electrophysiol 2008;31:1291–9.

2. Cronin EM, Ching EA, Varma N, et al. Remote monitoring of cardiovascular devices: a time and activity analysis. Heart Rhythm 2012;9(12):1947–51.

3. Crossley GH, Boyle A, Vitense H, et al. The CONNECT (Clinical Evaluation of Remote Notification to Reduce Time to Clinical Decision) trial: the value of wireless remote monitoring with automatic clinician alerts. J Am Coll Cardiol 2011;57: 1181–9.

4. Varma N, Epstein AE, Irimpen A, et al. Efficacy and safety of automatic remote monitoring for implantable cardioverter-defibrillator follow-up: the Lumos-T Safely Reduces Routine Office Device Follow-up (TRUST) trial. Circulation 2010;122:325–32.

5. Varma N, Stambler B, Chun S. Detection of atrial fibrillation by implanted devices with wireless data transmission capability. Pacing Clin Electrophysiol 2005;28(Suppl 1):S133–6.

6. Varma N, Pavri BB, Stambler B, et al. Same-day discovery of implantable cardioverter defibrillator dysfunction in the TRUST remote monitoring trial: influence of contrasting messaging systems. Europace 2013;15(5):697–703.

7. Mabo P, Victor F, Bazin P, et al. A randomized trial of long-term remote monitoring of pacemaker recipients (The COMPAS trial). Eur Heart J 2012;33: 1105–11.

8. Brignole M, Vardas P, Hoffman E, et al. Indications for the use of diagnostic implantable and external ECG loop recorders. Europace 2009;11:671–87.

9. Eitel C, Husser D, Hindricks G, et al. Performance of an implantable automatic atrial fibrillation detection device: impact of software adjustments and relevance of manual episode analysis. Europace 2011; 13:480–5.

10. Furukawa T, Maggi R, Bertolone C, et al. Effectiveness of remote monitoring in the management of syncope and palpitations. Europace 2011;13: 431–7.

11. Moya A, Sutton R, Ammirati F, et al. Guidelines for the diagnosis and management of syncope (version 2009): the Task Force for the Diagnosis and Management of Syncope of the European Society of Cardiology (ESC). Eur Heart J 2009;30:2631–71.

12. Brignole M, Sutton R, Menozzi C, et al. Early application of an implantable loop recorder allows effective specific therapy in patients with recurrent suspected neurally mediated syncope. Eur Heart J 2006;27: 1085–92.

13. Krahn AD, Klein GJ, Norris C, et al. The etiology of syncope in patients with negative tilt table and electrophysiological testing. Circulation 1995;92: 1819–24.

14. Paruchuri V, Adhaduk M, Garikipati NV, et al. Clinical utility of a novel wireless implantable loop recorder in the evaluation of patients with unexplained syncope. Heart Rhythm 2011;8:858–63.

15. Varma N, Michalski J, Epstein AE, et al. Automatic remote monitoring of implantable cardioverter-defibrillator lead and generator performance/clinical perspective. Circulation 2010;3:428–36.

16. Spencker S, Coban N, Koch L, et al. Potential role of home monitoring to reduce inappropriate shocks in implantable cardioverter-defibrillator patients due to lead failure. Europace 2009;11:483–8.

17. Ricci RP, Morichelli L, Gargaro A, et al. Home monitoring in patients with implantable cardiac devices: is there a potential reduction of stroke risk? Results from a computer model tested through Monte Carlo simulations. J Cardiovasc Electrophysiol 2009;20:1244–51.

18. The IMPACT of BIOTRONIK Home Monitoring Guided Anticoagulation on Stroke Risk in Patients With Implanted ICD and CRT-D Devices (IMPACT). Available at: http://www.clinicaltrials.gov/ct2/show/ NCT00559988. Accessed February 22, 2009.

19. Hindricks G, Piorkowski C, Tanner H, et al. Perception of atrial fibrillation before and after radiofrequency catheter ablation: relevance of asymptomatic arrhythmia recurrence. Circulation 2005;112:307–13.

20. Hindricks G, Pokushalov E, Urban L, et al. Performance of a new leadless implantable cardiac monitor in detecting and quantifying atrial fibrillation results of the XPECT trial. Circ Arrhythm Electrophysiol 2010;3:141–7.

21. Available at: http://clinicaltrials.gov/ct2/show/ NCT01061125. Accessed June 19, 2013.

22. Abraham WT, Adamson PB, Bourge RC, et al. Wireless pulmonary artery haemodynamic monitoring in chronic heart failure: a randomised controlled trial. Lancet 2011;377:658–66.

23. Whellan DJ, Ousdigian KT, Al-Khatib SM, et al. Combined heart failure device diagnostics identify patients at higher risk of subsequent heart failure hospitalizations: results from PARTNERS HF (Program to Access and Review Trending Information and Evaluate Correlation to Symptoms in Patients With Heart Failure) study. J Am Coll Cardiol 2010; 55:1803–10.

24. Mullens W, Grimm RA, Verga T, et al. Insights from a cardiac resynchronization optimization clinic as part of a heart failure disease management program. J Am Coll Cardiol 2009;53:765–73.

25. Saxon LA, Hayes DL, Gilliam FR, et al. Long-term outcome after ICD and CRT implantation and influence of remote device follow-up: the ALTITUDE survival study. Circulation 2010;122:2359–67.

26. Fischell TA, Fischell DR, Avezum A, et al. Initial clinical results using intracardiac electrogram monitoring to detect and alert patients during coronary plaque rupture and ischemia. J Am Coll Cardiol 2010;56:1089–98.

27. Forleo GB, Tesauro M, Panattoni G, et al. Impact of continuous intracardiac ST-segment monitoring on mid-term outcomes of ICD-implanted patients with

coronary artery disease. Early results of a prospective comparison with conventional ICD outcomes. Heart (British Cardiac Society) 2012;98:402–7.

28. Mabo P, Defaye P, Sadoul N, et al. Remote follow-up of patients implanted with and ICD: the prospective randomized EVATEL study. The European Society of Cardiology annual scientific sessions. 2011. http://spo.escardio.org/eslides/view.aspx?eevtid=48&fp=2173.

29. Varma N, Johnson MA. Prevalence of cancelled shock therapy and relationship to shock delivery in recipients of implantable cardioverter-defibrillators assessed by remote monitoring. Pacing Clin Electrophysiol 2009;32(Suppl 1):S42–6.

30. Guedon-Moreau L, Lacroix D, Sadoul N, et al. A randomized study of remote follow-up of implantable cardioverter defibrillators: safety and efficacy report of the ECOST trial. Eur Heart J 2013;34(8): 605–14.

31. Poole JE, Gleva MJ, Mela T, et al. Complication rates associated with pacemaker or implantable cardioverter-defibrillator generator replacements and upgrade procedures: results from the REPLACE registry. Circulation 2010;122:1553–61.

32. Varma N, Ricci RP. Telemedicine and cardiac implants: what is the benefit? Eur Heart J 2013. http://dx.doi.org/10.1093/eurheartj/ehs388. [Epub ahead of print].

Prolonged Rhythm Monitoring in the Patient with Stroke and Transient Ischemic Attack

Raymond C.S. Seet, MD[a,*], Alejandro A. Rabinstein, MD[b]

KEYWORDS

- Remote monitoring • Paroxysmal atrial fibrillation • Stroke • Transient ischemic attack

KEY POINTS

- Stroke patients undergo prolonged cardiac monitoring based on concern that those currently classified as having a cryptogenic cause and treated with antiplatelet therapy may actually have paroxysmal atrial fibrillation and merit anticoagulation for secondary stroke prevention.
- Technological advances have produced monitoring devices that can be applied to any patient, are capable of capturing electrocardiogram information accurately and continuously, and can relay critical data to the physician promptly and without the need for patient participation.
- Even if it is assumed that monitors can detect arrhythmias with perfect accuracy, it has yet to be demonstrated in clinical trials that more strokes can be prevented by anticoagulation guided by the findings of prolonged rhythm monitoring.
- As newer monitoring technology and safer anticoagulants continue to become available, clinical trials need to be conducted to determine the best clinical practice for stroke prevention in this rapidly evolving field.

INTRODUCTION

Atrial fibrillation (AF) is the most common sustained cardiac arrhythmia that is increasing in prevalence and incidence.[1] Over the past 2 decades, the incidence of AF has risen by 12.6% and, by 2050, 15.9 million individuals are projected to harbor AF.[1] Data from the Screening for Atrial Fibrillation in the Elderly study showed a prevalence of AF of 7.2% in patients aged 65 years and older, with an increased prevalence in men.[2] The attributable risk of stroke for AF increases with age, from 1.5% for those aged 50 to 59 years to 23.5% for those aged 80 to 89 years.[3] Strokes caused by AF are more disabling and fatal than strokes due to other causes, partly because occlusions caused by embolism tend to affect larger cerebral arteries, and partly because patients with AF -related stroke tend to be older than other patients with stroke, with multiple comorbidities, such as congestive heart failure, hypertension, and diabetes mellitus.[4]

AF is marked by the loss of coordinated atrial electrical and mechanical function and can be asymptomatic.[5,6] Reliance on symptoms to identify may significantly underestimate the prevalence of AF as asymptomatic AF occurs more than 12 times as often as symptomatic episodes when patients are followed up longitudinally by Holter monitoring.[7] Symptoms vary widely in the individual AF patient, from an incidental finding of palpitations and breathlessness on exercise to overt heart failure. Subclinical AF is not benign

Disclosures: Dr Seet receives grants from the National Medical Research Council and National Research Foundation, Singapore. Dr Rabinstein has received research support from CardioNet, Inc. and serves as safety monitor for a clinical trial funded by Boston Scientific.
[a] Department of Medicine, Yong Loo Lin School of Medicine, National University of Singapore, Singapore;
[b] Department of Neurology, Mayo Clinic, Rochester, MN, USA
* Corresponding author.
E-mail address: raymond_seet@nus.edu.sg

cardiacEP.theclinics.com

and is associated with at least the same risk for stroke as is symptomatic AF.[5] In some patients, a presentation with an AF-associated complication (eg, stroke or heart failure) might be the first manifestation of the arrhythmia. Traditionally, screening for AF in the community setting is limited to opportunistic clinical examination and electrocardiogram (ECG) monitoring. Although AF increases the risk of stroke by five-fold, this risk is not homogeneous and changes cumulatively with the presence of stroke risk factors.[8,9] These risk factors have been used to formulate various stroke risk stratification schema (**Tables 1** and **2**).[9]

AF, especially when paroxysmally present, can escape diagnosis. Paroxysmal AF comprises between 35% and 66% of all cases of AF and is defined as intermittent periods of AF interspersed with episodes of normal sinus rhythm. By contrast, persistent AF is diagnosed when an episode of AF either lasts longer than 7 days or needs

Table 1
CHADS$_2$ score and stroke rates

(a) Risk Factor-based Approach Expressed as a Point-based Scoring System, with the Acronym CHADS$_2$[a]

Risk Factor	Score
Congestive heart failure/ LV dysfunction	1
Hypertension	1
Age ≥75	1
Diabetes mellitus	1
Stroke/TIA/ thromboembolism	2
Maximum score	6

(b) Adjusted Stroke Rate according to CHADS$_2$ Score

CHADS$_2$ Score	Adjusted Stroke Risk (%/y)
0	1.9
1	2.8
2	4.0
3	5.9
4	8.5
5	12.5
6	18.2

Abbreviations: LV, left ventricular; TIA, transient ischemic attack.
[a] Maximum score is 6.
Data from Gage BF, Waterman AD, Shannon W, et al. Validation of clinical classification schemes for predicting stroke: results from the National Registry of Atrial Fibrillation. JAMA 2001;285(22):2867.

Table 2
CHA$_2$DS$_2$VASc score and stroke rates

(a) Risk Factor-based Approach Expressed as a Point-based Scoring System, with the Acronym CHA$_2$DS$_2$-VASc[a]

Risk Factor	Score
Congestive heart failure/ LV dysfunction	1
Hypertension	1
Age ≥75	2
Diabetes mellitus	1
Stroke/TIA/ thromboembolism	2
Vascular disease[b]	1
Age 65–74	1
Sex category (ie, female sex)	1
Maximum score	9

(b) Adjusted Stroke Rate according to CHA$_2$DS$_2$-VASc Score

CHA$_2$DS$_2$-VASc Score	Adjusted Stroke Risk (%/y)
0	0
1	1.3
2	2.2
3	3.2
4	4.0
5	6.7
6	9.8
7	9.6
8	6.7
9	15.2

Abbreviations: LV, left ventricular; TIA, transient ischemic attack.
[a] Maximum score is 9 because age may contribute 0, 1, or 2 points.
[b] Prior myocardial infarction, peripheral artery disease, aortic plaque. Actual rates of stroke in contemporary cohorts may vary from these estimates.
From Lip GY, Frison L, Halperin JL, et al. Comparative validation of a novel risk score for predicting bleeding risk in anticoagulated patients with atrial fibrillation: the HAS-BLED (Hypertension, Abnormal Renal/Liver Function, Stroke, Bleeding History or Predisposition, Labile INR, Elderly, Drugs/Alcohol Concomitantly) score. J Am Coll Cardiol 2011;57(2):177; with permission.

cardioversion, whereas longstanding persistent AF is considered when AF has lasted for 1 year or more and when a rhythm control strategy is used. Data from the Virtual International Stroke Trials Archive indicate delayed detection of AF in approximately 7% of stroke patients.[10] In most of these patients, AF was detected more than

48 hours after presentation.[10] In patients with paroxysmal AF determined by standard surface ECG tracings, the risk of stroke in patients with paroxysmal AF is similar to that observed with chronic and persistent forms of AF[11] and current guidelines recommend treating paroxysmal AF based on the concomitant stroke risk factors in a manner identical to persistent forms with regards to stroke prophylaxis.[12,13]

With improvements in technology, there is expanding interest to develop newer cardiac monitoring devices that are easy to wear and sufficiently small to hide under most clothing, thus allowing for prolonged monitoring.[14] In unselected populations, new paroxysmal AF (diagnosed using inpatient and/or ambulatory ECG devices) is observed in 5% of stroke and transient ischemic attack patients.[14] However, when more stringent criteria are applied (based on suspected stroke cause and age), the detection rate increases to 11%.[14] Not surprisingly, studies that monitored patients for a longer period identified a higher incidence of AF.[14] These devices are capable of rigorously defining the AF burden as the measured percentage of time spent in AF during the follow-up period. AF burden is a parameter that takes into account the frequency and duration of AF episodes during the overall follow-up period, and daily AF burden is an estimate of the overall duration of AF episodes in each day. The trend of daily AF burden during the follow-up period is an easy and efficient way to show the presence and evolution of the disease.

Data from a large-scale pacemaker trial, Asymptomatic Atrial Fibrillation and Stroke Evaluation in Pacemaker Patients and the Atrial Fibrillation Reduction Atrial Pacing Trial (ASSERT) further underscore the usefulness of cardiac rhythm monitoring.[15] In this study, patients were classified with and without AF through the diagnostics of the implanted pacemakers. Patients were defined as free of AF if they did not have any AF episodes lasting more than 6 minutes. At 3 months, 10% of ASSERT patients had ≥ 1 AF episode lasting more than 6 minutes. AF, as detected by the implanted device, was associated with a 2.5-fold increased risk of ischemic stroke and systemic embolism, confirming the clinical value of implantable devices.[15]

CARDIAC RHYTHM MONITORING

For an assessment of a patient with AF, confirmation of the diagnosis and documentation of the arrhythmia are needed. An irregular pulse may raise suspicion for AF but the gold standard for diagnosing AF remains the visual inspection of a 12-lead ECG. Guidelines from the American Heart Association and the European Society of Cardiology (ESC) define AF as a cardiac arrhythmia with the following characteristics: the surface ECG shows absolutely irregular R-R intervals; there are no distinct P waves on the surface ECG; and the atrial cycle length (ie, the interval between 2 atrial activations), when visible, is usually variable and less than 200 ms (>300 beats/min).[13] A standard 12-lead ECG can also indicate alternative causes of arrhythmia, such as the pre-excitation in Wolff-Parkinson-White syndrome, inherited cardiac arrhythmic syndromes (eg, long QT and Brugada syndrome), inherited cardiomyopathic syndrome (eg, atrioventricular block), and hypertrophic cardiomyopathy.

Arrhythmias can be paroxysmal and asymptomatic. Thus, a baseline resting ECG may be insufficient for diagnosis. In practice, the optimal method of cardiac monitoring to detect these paroxysmal arrhythmias depends largely on the availability of devices and relevant expertise, cost considerations, convenience, and acceptability to patients as well as the desired duration of monitoring. Since the development of the Holter monitor in the 1940s, there has been progressive development in cardiac rhythm monitoring technology. Numerous cardiac devices have become available to detect paroxysmal AF; these devices are capable of distinguishing AF from other arrhythmias and to monitor its response to antiarrhythmic treatments.[14] AF detection devices are divided into the 3 following categories: (1) surface ECG systems; (2) subcutaneous recording systems; and (3) intracardiac recording systems.

Surface Recording Systems

During Holter monitoring, a patient is typically connected to 3 to 5 ECG electrodes, which yield 2 ECG vectors and a third derived electrocardiogram. The patient maintains a diary to document the time when symptoms are experienced and their description. After the 1- to 2-day recording period is completed, the patient returns the monitor; the data stored within the electronic media are downloaded to a local workstation or transmitted over the Internet to a central workstation. The computer-scanned Holter recording is read by a trained technician who then forwards the report to the physician for final review and interpretation. Assuming that the recording quality is adequate, Holter monitors can determine the average heart rate and heart rate range, quantify atrial and ventricular ectopy counts, and determine whether AF is present. Information on the shortest and longest duration of AF, burden of

AF, the heart rate during AF, and pattern of initiation and termination of AF can also be determined. Many recorders include patient-activated event markers as well as time markers to allow better correlation between symptoms and rhythm abnormalities. The major limitation of Holter monitoring, however, is the relatively short recording period, typically 1 to 2 days.

Patient-activated event recorders can be used for several weeks at a time. Event recorders are small, leadless devices that are carried by the patient. When a patient experiences a symptom, the device is applied to the chest wall. Because electrodes are present on the back of the device, a brief (typically up to 90 s) single-lead ECG recording can be stored. The event recorder can store only a few tracings because they have only about 10 minutes of storage capacity; thus, to minimize loss of data, once an event is recorded, it needs to be immediately transmitted transtelephonically (ie, transmitting recordings by telephone by converting ECG data to audio signals) to a central monitoring site for validation and analysis. By design, event recorders do not provide information about asymptomatic episodes. These event recorders are useful for symptomatic patients and are typically tolerated up to 4 weeks in motivated patients.

Ambulatory telemetry monitoring was developed to overcome many of the limitations inherent to Holter and event and event recorders, namely, the need for long-term monitoring and the ability to capture information about symptomatic and asymptomatic arrhythmias. Typically, patients are connected by 3 or 4 ECG electrodes to a battery-powered sensor for up to 30 days. The sensor can hold anywhere from 6 hours to 30 days of ECG data. Data from the sensor are sent to the handheld device when it is within 10 to 300 ft of the patient. Once the patient is in a location with available cellular coverage, the stored ECG data are transmitted from the handheld device to a central monitoring station. If a patient travels outside of the cellular network, data are stored and transmitted when back in range. Patients can also use the handheld device to enter information about symptoms. The monitoring center can determine whether the patient is actually wearing the device and ascertain the quality of the contact with the ECG electrodes; by communicating directly with the patient, compliance with the system and quality of the acquired data may be improved.

Subcutaneous Recording Systems

Implantable loop recorders are small (typically 6 cm × 2 cm × 0.8 cm) devices implanted subcutaneously to overcome the limitations of skin irritation and patient compliance and allow very prolonged recording periods. They automatically record tachyarrhythmias and bradyarrhythmias with programmable parameters or when a patient triggers a recording with a wireless activator. The duration and number of recordings are programmable, with current devices capable of recording up to 50 minutes of ECG. Data can be transmitted over the telephone or wirelessly with appropriate equipment to the Internet for web-based physician review. The implant may be left in place up to 3 years and can be explanted once a diagnosis is made or the battery life has ended. Automatic triggers and the lack of external electrodes minimize the need for patient compliance to capture an event.

Intracardiac Recording Systems

In contrast to surface and subcutaneous systems, dual-chamber pacemakers and implantable cardioverter-defibrillators detect atrial tachyarrhythmias with a regular ventricular response, even if the ventricular rate is in the normal range. By contrast, single-chamber implantable cardioverter-defibrillators only detect arrhythmias if the ventricular rate exceeds the ventricular tachycardia detection rate. Thus, for reliable detection of atrial arrhythmias, dual-chamber systems are often used. Cardiac implantable electronic device batteries last 5 to 12 years, depending on the device type and therapy delivered.

SIGNIFICANCE OF AF BURDEN

Cardiac rhythm monitoring devices are capable of identifying very brief episodes of paroxysmal AF (even lasting for a few seconds), the significance of which is uncertain. Existing data suggest that not all atrial tachyarrhythmias are the same and that AF duration and frequency of recurrence are probably important clinical parameters when measured using a reliable technique. Glotzer and colleagues[16] showed that patients with atrial arrhythmias defined as atrial arrhythmias lasting more than 5 minutes had a 5.9 times greater chance of developing clinical AF and a 2.8 times greater risk for stroke or death. Capucci and colleagues[17] showed that the risk for embolism, adjusted for known risk factors, was 3.1 times increased in patients with device-detected AF episodes greater than 1 day during follow-up. In the Prospective Study of the Clinical Significance of Atrial Arrhythmias Detected by Implanted Device Diagnostics trial, the median daily AF burden was 5.5 hours in 1 of the 30 days preceding a stroke or transient ischemic attack.[18] When the daily burden was greater than 5.5 hours, the patient had a 2.4 greater risk for stroke compared with patients with lower daily burdens.[18] There are suggestions that adding data of daily AF burden can improve risk stratification for stroke when either the CHADS$_2$ or the CHA$_2$DS$_2$VASc score is used.[19]

PATIENT SELECTION

In stroke and transient ischemic attack patients, the detection yield for AF is improved when selection criteria for prolonged cardiac monitoring is applied. In previous analyses, patients were selected based on their age, stroke subtypes, stroke location, and clinical stroke severity. Twenty-five percent of ischemic strokes remain unexplained after an initial thorough evaluation (including 12-lead ECG and in-hospital telemetry monitoring) and are designated cryptogenic stroke. Strokes related to AF are associated with an approximately 50% increased risk of disability and 60% increased risk of death at 3 months compared with strokes of other causes.[3] A higher incidence of AF was observed in patients with cryptogenic stroke as compared with those with large atherothrombotic and lacunar strokes in one study.[20] It is thought that cardiogenic embolism due to undetected paroxysmal AF is probably responsible for a substantial part of cryptogenic ischemic strokes. Studies restricted to patients with cryptogenic stroke found an incidence of AF ranging between 14.3% and 27.3%.[21–23] In younger patients with cryptogenic stroke, however, the use of implantable loop recorders was not able to detect new cases of AF.[24] Among patients with suspected embolic strokes, the incidence of AF was 6% in one study that used a 72-hour ambulatory ECG monitoring device.[25] The ongoing study Study of Continuous Cardiac Monitoring to Assess Atrial Fibrillation After Cryptogenic Stroke is investigating the value of even longer term monitoring using an implantable loop recorder, emphasizing the importance of identifying which patients with cryptogenic stroke should be candidates for anticoagulation.[26]

Because an embolus from the heart may preferentially lodge in the anterior circulation, or break up and lead to multiple ischemic foci, studies assessing infarcted territory and its association with AF have been performed. **Fig. 1** describes radiological patterns of cardioembolic stroke. In one study, the incidence of AF was higher in patients with anterior circulation territory infarctions than in those with lacunar stroke (68% vs 0%).[27] Patients with AF had more often severe neurologic deficits (National Institute of Health Stroke Scale >10) compared with those without AF

(n = 5, 22.7% vs n = 4, 3.1%, P = .003).[27] In other studies, neuroimaging parameters, such as infarct size,[21] number of infarcts,[28] and stroke locations,[29,30] were identified as significant predictors of AF detection after an acute stroke. A combination of clinical and radiological features (comprising embolic infarct pattern, age >65 years, and pre-existent coronary artery disease) has been also associated with a higher incidence of AF.[30] There is increasing consensus that prolonged cardiac monitoring should be reserved for selected patients with cryptogenic stroke and cerebrovascular events suspicious for embolism.

CLINICAL PERSPECTIVE

Continuous monitoring is a powerful tool to detect silent paroxysmal AF in patients without previously documented arrhythmic episodes, such as those with cryptogenic stroke or other risk factors. Early diagnosis would trigger early treatment for secondary stroke prevention.

Central to the successful management of AF is the early identification and treatment of predisposing factors and concomitant disorders, with the use of angiotensin-converting enzyme inhibitors, angiotensin-receptor blockers, statins, and ω-3 polyunsaturated fatty acids, when appropriate.[13] A prothrombotic state has been described in atrial fibrillation, and it contributes to the most important complication of thromboembolism.[31] Randomized trials have shown that warfarin is highly effective in preventing stroke in patients with AF, most likely by minimizing the formation of atrial thrombi.[32,33] Management guidelines have traditionally recommended that high-risk patients be given oral anticoagulation, whereas patients at moderate (or intermediate) risk can be treated with oral anticoagulation or aspirin, and low-risk patients with aspirin. In fact, the most recent guidelines from the American College of Chest Physicians have lowered the threshold to recommend oral anticoagulation in patients with paroxysmal AF.[34] In a meta-analysis by Hart and colleagues,[33] adjusted dose warfarin reduced stroke risk by 64% (95% confidence interval 49–74) and, importantly, all-cause mortality by 26% (3–43) compared with placebo. Oral anticoagulation was associated with a 39% (95% confidence interval 22–50) risk reduction compared with antiplatelet therapy, which provides indirect evidence that antiplatelet therapy could be very modestly effective for stroke prevention.[33] Findings from the Atrial fibrillation Clopidogrel Trial with Irbesartan for prevention of Vascular Events (ACTIVE-W) trial showed a clear superiority of warfarin over aspirin plus clopidogrel combination therapy for stroke

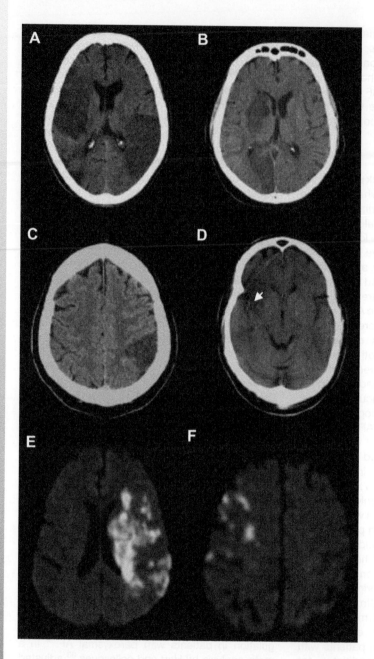

Fig. 1. Radiological patterns of cardioembolic stroke. (A) Head computed tomography (CT) scan showing bilateral ischemic infarctions. (B) CT scan showing brain infarctions in 2 different vascular territories (middle cerebral artery in the anterior circulation and posterior cerebral artery in the posterior circulation). (C) CT scan illustrating a characteristic wedge-shaped embolic infarction based in the cortex. (D) CT scan displaying a cortical infarction in the right frontal lobe in association with a hyperdense intravascular signal in an M2 segment of the right middle cerebral artery indicates an acute occluding clot (arrow). (E) Diffusion-weighted imaging sequence of a brain magnetic resonance imaging scan demonstrating scattered areas of restricted diffusion in the left middle cerebral artery distribution indicative of acute ischemia. (F) Diffusion-weighted imaging magnetic resonance imaging showing multiple small areas of brain infarction in a pattern consistent with an "embolic shower." (From Rabinstein AA, Resnick SJ. Practical neuroimaging in stroke. Philadelphia, PA: Saunders Elsevier; 2009; with permission.)

prevention.[35] Furthermore, aspirin plus clopidogrel reduced the rate of ischemic stroke by 28% compared with aspirin alone.[36]

Because paroxysmal AF is as likely as continuous AF to increase the risk of recurrent stroke,[10,33] it seems logical to extrapolate the significance of these brief episodes of AF detected by prolonged rhythm monitoring to traditional definitions of paroxysmal AF (ie, intermittent periods of AF interspersed with episodes of normal sinus rhythm documented by conventional electrocardiography) and to assume the same benefits of

long-term anticoagulation in these cases, which becomes especially relevant now that the availability of new and safer oral anticoagulant drugs that do not need monitoring provide more enticing options for thromboprophylaxis in AF. However, it is necessary to exercise caution when making these assumptions because the threshold of AF burden above which the benefits of anticoagulation outweighs its bleeding risk remains unclear. How much paroxysmal AF detected by prolonged rhythm monitoring should be present to warrant anticoagulation for stroke prevention? In a patient with cryptogenic stroke, is a single episode of paroxysmal AF for a few minutes sufficient to prescribe anticoagulation, knowing that paroxysmal AF is so prevalent and may also be detected by prolonged rhythm monitoring in patients with comparable risk factors but without stroke? What if the isolated episode of AF only lasts a few seconds over a long period of monitoring? These questions are even more pertinent because cerebral infarction in itself (especially when involving the insular cortex) has been reported to be a cause of cardiac rhythm abnormalities.[37,38]

To date, there are no data from randomized controlled trials to guide the appropriate treatment of brief episodes of paroxysmal AF detected by prolonged rhythm monitoring. The IMPACT trial will attempt to provide some answers to this important clinical question.[39]

SUMMARY

The impetus for prolonged cardiac monitoring in stroke patients stems from concerns that cases currently classified as cryptogenic and treated with antiplatelet therapy may actually have paroxysmal AF and merit anticoagulation for secondary stroke prevention. In this regard, technological advances have produced monitoring devices that can be applied to any patient, are capable of capturing ECG information accurately and continuously, and can relay critical data to the physician promptly and without the need for patient participation. However, even if it is assumed that these monitors can detect arrhythmias with perfect accuracy, it has yet to be demonstrated in clinical trials that more strokes can be prevented by anticoagulation guided by the findings of prolonged rhythm monitoring. As newer monitoring technology and safer anticoagulants continue to become available, clinical trials need to be conducted to determine the best clinical practice for stroke prevention in this rapidly evolving field.

REFERENCES

1. Miyasaka Y, Barnes ME, Gersh BJ, et al. Secular trends in incidence of atrial fibrillation in Olmsted County, Minnesota, 1980 to 2000, and implications on the projections for future prevalence. Circulation 2006;114:119–25.
2. Hobbs FD, Fitzmaurice DA, Mant J, et al. A randomised controlled trial and cost-effectiveness study of systematic screening (targeted and total population screening) versus routine practice for the detection of atrial fibrillation in people aged 65 and over. The SAFE study. Health Technol Assess 2005;9:iii–iv, ix–x, 1–74.
3. Wolf PA, Abbott RD, Kannel WB. Atrial fibrillation as an independent risk factor for stroke: the Framingham study. Stroke 1991;22:983–8.
4. Gattellari M, Goumas C, Aitken R, et al. Outcomes for patients with ischaemic stroke and atrial fibrillation: the PRISM study (a Program of Research Informing Stroke Management). Cerebrovasc Dis 2011;32:370–82.
5. Flaker GC, Belew K, Beckman K, et al. Asymptomatic atrial fibrillation: demographic features and prognostic information from the atrial fibrillation follow-up investigation of rhythm management (AFFIRM) study. Am Heart J 2005;149:657–63.
6. Israel CW, Gronefeld G, Ehrlich JR, et al. Long-term risk of recurrent atrial fibrillation as documented by an implantable monitoring device: implications for optimal patient care. J Am Coll Cardiol 2004;43:47–52.
7. Page RL, Wilkinson WE, Clair WK, et al. Asymptomatic arrhythmias in patients with symptomatic paroxysmal atrial fibrillation and paroxysmal supraventricular tachycardia. Circulation 1994;89:224–7.
8. Stroke Risk in Atrial Fibrillation Working Group. Independent predictors of stroke in patients with atrial fibrillation: a systematic review. Neurology 2007;69:546–54.
9. Hughes M, Lip GY. Stroke and thromboembolism in atrial fibrillation: a systematic review of stroke risk factors, risk stratification schema and cost effectiveness data. Thromb Haemost 2008;99:295–304.
10. Kamel H, Lees KR, Lyden PD, et al. Delayed detection of atrial fibrillation after ischemic stroke. J Stroke Cerebrovasc Dis 2009;18:453–7.
11. Friberg L, Hammar N, Rosenqvist M. Stroke in paroxysmal atrial fibrillation: report from the Stockholm cohort of atrial fibrillation. Eur Heart J 2010;31:967–75.
12. Fuster V, Ryden LE, Cannom DS, et al. ACC/AHA/ESC 2006 Guidelines for the Management of patients with Atrial Fibrillation-Executive Summary: a report of the American College of Cardiology/American Heart Association task force on practice guidelines and the European Society of Cardiology committee for practice guidelines (writing committee to revise the 2001 guidelines for the management of patients with atrial fibrillation). Eur Heart J 2006;27:1979–2030.
13. Camm AJ, Kirchhof P, Lip GY, et al. Guidelines for the management of atrial fibrillation: the task force for the management of atrial fibrillation of the European Society of Cardiology (ESC). Eur Heart J 2010;31:2369–429.
14. Seet RC, Friedman PA, Rabinstein AA. Prolonged rhythm monitoring for the detection of occult paroxysmal atrial fibrillation in ischemic stroke of unknown cause. Circulation 2011;124:477–86.

15. Healey JS, Connolly SJ, Gold MR, et al. Subclinical atrial fibrillation and the risk of stroke. N Engl J Med 2012;366:120–9.

16. Glotzer TV, Hellkamp AS, Zimmerman J, et al. Atrial high rate episodes detected by pacemaker diagnostics predict death and stroke: report of the Atrial Diagnostics Ancillary Study of the Mode Selection trial (MOST). Circulation 2003;107:1614–9.

17. Capucci A, Santini M, Padeletti L, et al. Monitored atrial fibrillation duration predicts arterial embolic events in patients suffering from bradycardia and atrial fibrillation implanted with antitachycardia pacemakers. J Am Coll Cardiol 2005;46:1913–20.

18. Glotzer TV, Daoud EG, Wyse DG, et al. The relationship between daily atrial tachyarrhythmia burden from implantable device diagnostics and stroke risk: the TRENDS study. Circ Arrhythm Electrophysiol 2009;2:474–80.

19. Boriani G, Botto GL, Padeletti L, et al. Improving stroke risk stratification using the $CHADS_2$ and CHA_2DS_2-VASC risk scores in patients with paroxysmal atrial fibrillation by continuous arrhythmia burden monitoring. Stroke 2011;42:1768–70.

20. Shafqat S, Kelly PJ, Furie KL. Holter monitoring in the diagnosis of stroke mechanism. Intern Med J 2004;34:305–9.

21. Sposato LA, Klein FR, Jauregui A, et al. Newly diagnosed atrial fibrillation after acute ischemic stroke and transient ischemic attack: importance of immediate and prolonged continuous cardiac monitoring. J Stroke Cerebrovasc Dis 2012;21:210–6.

22. Elijovich L, Josephson SA, Fung GL, et al. Intermittent atrial fibrillation may account for a large proportion of otherwise cryptogenic stroke: a study of 30-day cardiac event monitors. J Stroke Cerebrovasc Dis 2009;18:185–9.

23. Barthelemy JC, Feasson-Gerard S, Garnier P, et al. Automatic cardiac event recorders reveal paroxysmal atrial fibrillation after unexplained strokes or transient ischemic attacks. Ann Noninvasive Electrocardiol 2003;8:194–9.

24. Dion F, Saudeau D, Bonnaud I, et al. Unexpected low prevalence of atrial fibrillation in cryptogenic ischemic stroke: a prospective study. J Interv Card Electrophysiol 2010;28:101–7.

25. Schuchert A, Behrens G, Meinertz T. Impact of long-term ECG recording on the detection of paroxysmal atrial fibrillation in patients after an acute ischemic stroke. Pacing Clin Electrophysiol 1999;22:1082–4.

26. Sinha AM, Diener HC, Morillo CA, et al. Cryptogenic stroke and underlying atrial fibrillation (CRYSTAL AF): design and rationale. Am Heart J 2010;160:36–41.

27. Jabaudon D, Sztajzel J, Sievert K, et al. Usefulness of ambulatory 7-day ECG monitoring for the detection of atrial fibrillation and flutter after acute stroke and transient ischemic attack. Stroke 2004; 35:1647–51.

28. Alhadramy O, Jeerakathil TJ, Majumdar SR, et al. Prevalence and predictors of paroxysmal atrial fibrillation on Holter monitor in patients with stroke or transient ischemic attack. Stroke 2010;41:2596–600.

29. Gaillard N, Deltour S, Vilotijevic B, et al. Detection of paroxysmal atrial fibrillation with transtelephonic EKG in TIA or stroke patients. Neurology 2010;74: 1666–70.

30. Lazzaro MA, Krishnan K, Prabhakaran S. Detection of atrial fibrillation with concurrent Holter monitoring and continuous cardiac telemetry following ischemic stroke and transient ischemic attack. J Stroke Cerebrovasc Dis 2012;21:89–93.

31. Watson T, Shantsila E, Lip GY. Mechanisms of thrombogenesis in atrial fibrillation: Virchow's triad revisited. Lancet 2009;373:155–66.

32. Manning WJ, Silverman DI, Waksmonski CA, et al. Prevalence of residual left atrial thrombi among patients with acute thromboembolism and newly recognized atrial fibrillation. Arch Intern Med 1995; 155:2193–8.

33. Hart RG, Benavente O, McBride R, et al. Antithrombotic therapy to prevent stroke in patients with atrial fibrillation: a meta-analysis. Ann Intern Med 1999; 131:492–501.

34. You JJ, Singer DE, Howard PA, et al. Antithrombotic therapy for atrial fibrillation: antithrombotic therapy and prevention of thrombosis, 9th ed: American College of Chest Physicians Evidence-based Clinical Practice Guidelines. Chest 2012;141:e531S–75S.

35. Connolly S, Pogue J, Hart R, et al. Clopidogrel plus aspirin versus oral anticoagulation for atrial fibrillation in the atrial fibrillation clopidogrel trial with irbesartan for prevention of vascular events (ACTIVE W): a randomised controlled trial. Lancet 2006;367: 1903–12.

36. Connolly SJ, Pogue J, Hart RG, et al. Effect of clopidogrel added to aspirin in patients with atrial fibrillation. N Engl J Med 2009;360:2066–78.

37. Oppenheimer S. Cerebrogenic cardiac arrhythmias: cortical lateralization and clinical significance. Clin Auton Res 2006;16:6–11.

38. Vingerhoets F, Bogousslavsky J, Regli F, et al. Atrial fibrillation after acute stroke. Stroke 1993;24:26–30.

39. Ip J, Waldo AL, Lip GY, et al. Multicenter randomized study of anticoagulation guided by remote rhythm monitoring in patients with implantable cardioverter-defibrillator and CRT-D devices: rationale, design, and clinical characteristics of the initially enrolled cohort the IMPACT study. Am Heart J 2009;158:364–70.

Remote Monitoring for Atrial Fibrillation

Jonathan P. Man, MD[a], Suraj Kapa, MD[b],
Sanjay Dixit, MD[a],*

KEYWORDS

- Atrial fibrillation • Remote monitoring • Ablation • Stroke

KEY POINTS

- The diagnostic yield of remote monitoring for atrial fibrillation (AF) improves with longer periods of monitoring, being greatest with monitored telemetry and least with short-term (24–48 hour) Holters.
- The burden of AF required to incur an increased risk of thromboembolic complications may range from 5 minutes to 24 hours.
- There is poor symptom-rhythm correlation in AF, and identifying episodes of AF is better with the use of monitoring rather than patient-reported symptoms alone.
- Monitoring to manage patients after prior AF ablation is useful to identify clinically significant arrhythmia recurrence, and implantable loop recorders (ILRs) may prove more useful than external monitoring strategies, such as transtelephonic monitors (TTMs) or monitored telemetry.

INTRODUCTION

AF is a common arrhythmia, with an estimated prevalence of 2.2 million people in the United States, and is responsible for approximately half a million hospitalizations yearly, with an estimated cost of approximately $7300 per discharge.[1] The risk of AF increases with age, with a lifetime risk of 25% for developing AF after the age of 40.[2] AF is also associated with increased morbidity, including ischemic stroke due to thromboembolic complications, heart failure, and death.[3–7]

One of the limitations in the diagnosis and management of AF, however, is the inability to identify the arrhythmia in patients without a prior history, to correlate the arrhythmia with symptoms and to recognize overall AF burden. AF is an independent risk factor for stroke and this risk may exist even with rare AF episodes as short as 5 minutes in duration and in the absence of associated symptoms.[3–7] Thus, monitoring for AF is key to caring for patients, whether in terms of initial diagnosis or ongoing treatment.

Traditionally, monitoring for AF may consist of cost-effective methods, such as daily or twice-daily pulse checks performed by patients. The other end of the spectrum comprises implantable monitors (eg, loop recorders) that may continuously record the heart rhythm over the course of years. The choice of monitoring strategy, however, needs to be tied to the clinical situation (eg, whether it is done for initial diagnosis or for evaluating treatment efficacy). This review focuses on the wide variety of remote monitoring options available for patients presenting with AF and the evidence surrounding their relative indications. Novel modalities that may offer benefit to managing patients with AF in the future are also discussed.

Disclosures: The author has nothing to disclose.
a Section of Cardiac Electrophysiology, Department of Medicine, Hospital of the University of Pennsylvania, 9 Founders Pavilion, 3400 Spruce Street, Philadelphia, PA 19104, USA; b Division of Cardiology, Mayo Clinic College of Medicine, 200 First Street SW, Rochester, MN 55905, USA
* Corresponding author.
E-mail address: Sanjay.Dixit@uphs.upenn.edu

Card Electrophysiol Clin 5 (2013) 357–364
http://dx.doi.org/10.1016/j.ccep.2013.05.008
1877-9182/13/$ – see front matter © 2013 Elsevier Inc. All rights reserved.

OPTIONS FOR MONITORING ATRIAL FIBRILLATION

Monitoring for AF has 3 goals: to determine if AF is present, to correlate symptoms with the underlying rhythm, and to evaluate the efficacy of drugs on the heart rate and AF burden. There are several different options for remote monitoring (**Table 1**).[8]

Holter monitoring allows monitoring a patient's heart rhythm for the period of time the monitor is worn (usually 24–72 hours). The data are stored on the device and interpreted after it is delivered back to the clinician's office. Disadvantages include the need to keep a symptom log and the size of the device, which is cumbersome to some patients.

Event recorders or TTMs are divided into continuous loop recorders and postevent monitors. Continuous loop recorders have leads attached to a patient, who can then trigger the device. The device also has automatic triggers that, in response to specific arrhythmias, store arrhythmia events that may not necessarily correlate with symptoms. There is a memory limit and the data must be transmitted manually or else it is overwritten. Postevent monitors are applied after an event and record the rhythm over the short period of time preceding the event. Advantages include smaller size and longer monitoring time. Postevent monitors rely, however, on a patient being able to apply the monitor and, thus, may miss short-lived events. Successful identification of arrhythmias with postevent monitors has been reported as approximately 60%, which is less than ideal, and this is likely because successful arrhythmia documentation requires the ability of a patient to apply the monitor, record the event, and then transmit the data.[9]

Real-time continuous monitoring, such as with a TTM, also relies on the application of leads to the body. Data are continuously transmitted and analyzed, however, and do not depend on a patient's ability to transmit data. The cost of TTM is much higher than for a Holter ($750 vs $275).[8] Monitored telemetry is yet another form of remote monitoring. During the monitoring period, the patient's heart rhythm is continuously watched by appropriately trained live personnel. Because this is more labor intensive, it is significantly more costly than other monitoring options.

ILRs are devices placed subcutaneously, thereby necessitating a surgical procedure to implant and remove them. They have the advantage of longer-term monitoring (up to 3 years) for rare events. Recordings are manually triggered by a patient or autotriggered when certain programmable parameters are met.

Finally, all dual-chamber pacemakers and defibrillators can record AF and transmit the information remotely. Pacemakers and defibrillators are implanted, however, for reasons other than to solely monitor AF and thus do not play a role as a stand-alone monitoring modality in patients with AF.

ATRIAL FIBRILLATION MANAGEMENT—ARE SYMPTOMS ENOUGH? EVIDENCE FOR USING REMOTE MONITORING IN DIAGNOSIS

Asymptomatic Atrial Fibrillation

Not all AF is symptomatic and up to 20% of AFs are found incidentally on routine clinical examination.[10,11] Studies on the use of monitors, such as Holter and TTMs, suggest that the incidence of asymptomatic AF may range from 20% to 30% in an otherwise healthy population.[12–14] One study of patients undergoing pacemaker implant showed the incidence of asymptomatic AF as high as 38%.[15] Clinically silent AF can have consequences, as seen in 2 large trials that compared the treatment strategies of rate versus rhythm control.[16,17] Patients randomized to rhythm control in both studies had a similar incidence of thromboembolic complications compared with patients

Table 1
Summary of remote monitoring options

Device	Duration of Monitoring	Complete Storage of Data (24/d)	Remote Transmission
Holter	1–2 d but up to 2 wk	Yes	No
Transtelephonic Monitor/Event Recorders			
Continuous loop	Up to 1 mo	No	Yes
Postevent (nonlooping)	Up to 1 mo	No	Yes
Real-time continuous monitoring	Up to 1 mo	Yes	Yes
ILR	Up to 2 y	No	Yes

Adapted from Zimetbaum P, Goldman A. Ambulatory arrhythmia monitoring: choosing the right device. Circulation 2010;122:1629–36; with permission.

randomized to rate control, even when presenting in sinus rhythm at the time of doctors' visits. The similar incidence of thromboembolism in these studies was attributed to asymptomatic AF. Thus, there is a large incidence of clinically asymptomatic AF and this incidence may not be entirely benign. Given these patients may present without symptoms, however, the only way to identify these patients is by using specific monitoring modalities, the choice of which needs to be guided by cost, patient context, and clinical suspicion.

Atrial Fibrillation Incidentally Discovered by Implanted Pacemakers/Defibrillators

Implanted cardiac rhythm management devices (pacemakers and defibrillators) continuously monitor patients' heart rhythms. Thus, even though these devices are implanted for other indications, they may be useful in evaluating for asymptomatic AF. This is supported by one study in which 110 patients with a history of either persistent or paroxysmal AF and a class I pacing indication were followed.[17] Fifty patients (45%) had AF recurrences, with 19 (38%) of them having asymptomatic AF. Despite 60 of 110 patients (55%) having 3 months free of AF, 23% (n = 14) of these patients later developed asymptomatic AF lasting over 48 hours. Symptom-rhythm correlation was poor, with as many as 44% (n = 48) of all patients reporting symptoms in the absence of AF.

The Relationship Between Daily Atrial Tachyarrhythmia Burden From Implantable Device Diagnostics and Stroke Risk (TRENDS) study examined the role of AF burden in risk of thromboembolic complications, such as stroke.[18] Atrial tachycardia (AT) and AF were defined in this study as an atrial rate greater than 175 beats per minute lasting 20 seconds or more. This study did not attempt to differentiate between AT or AF. Overall, 2813 patients were followed for a mean of 1.4 years. Patients with a low AT/AF burden (defined as <5.5 hours on each of 30 preceding days) had a thromboembolism risk similar to patients without any AT/AF (hazard ratio 0.98; 95% CI, 0.34–2.82; P = .97). Meanwhile, a high AT/AF burden (>5.5 hours on any given day during the 30 preceding days) seemed to double the risk of thromboembolic complications (hazard ratio 2.20; 95% CI, 0.96–5.05; P = .06). The investigators noted that

the overall lower-than-expected thromboembolism rate in this study made it difficult to accurately correlate thromboembolic risk with arrhythmia burden. Thus, they cautioned that because of the wide CIs, there may be no safe amount of AT/AF as far as thromboembolic risk is concerned.

One prospective trial (Asymptomatic Atrial Fibrillation and Stroke Evaluation in Pacemaker Patients and the Atrial Fibrillation Reduction Atrial Pacing Trial [ASSERT]) examined patients with no history of AF, who were 65 years or older with a history of hypertension and had an implantable cardiac defibrillator or pacemaker.[19] For 3 months the patients were monitored for subclinical atrial arrhythmias, which were defined as episodes of a rapid atrial rate of 190 beats or more per minute lasting more than 6 minutes detected by the pacemaker or defibrillator. These patients (n = 2580) were followed for a mean of 2.5 years. In the 3-month period, 10.1% (n = 261) of patients had a subclinical atrial arrhythmia with a median number of 2 episodes. Of those patients, 4.2% (n = 11) had a stroke with an annualized risk of 1.69% per year. This contrasted with those patients (n = 2319) without subclinical atrial arrhythmias who had an overall incidence of stroke of 1.7% (n = 40), with an annualized risk of 0.69% per year. The hazard ratio (2.50; 95% CI, 1.28–4.89; P = .008) between the 2 groups was virtually unchanged after controlling for other risk factors or when patients who went on to develop clinical AF were removed from the analysis. When patients were stratified according to atrial arrhythmia duration, the longest AF duration showed a statistically significant difference in annual stroke or thromboembolic risk for the longest episodes (Table 2). Of the 261 patients who had subclinical atrial arrhythmias, 15.7% (n = 41) went on to develop clinical atrial arrhythmias identified by ECG during routine clinic visits.

These studies on patients with previously implanted devices suggest that there is a high incidence of asymptomatic AF that may not be otherwise clinically recognizable and that, in turn, the presence of AF may cause an increased risk of stroke. The AF burden necessary to place somebody at increased risk of thromboembolic complications is, however, unclear. Other studies have tried to examine the relationship between AF burden and stroke risk. A subgroup analysis

Table 2
ASSERT data showing relationship between AF duration and annual stroke or embolic event

	≤0.86 h	0.87–3.63 h	3.64–17.72 h	>17.72 h
Annual rate (95% CI)	1.23 (0.15–4.46)	0 (0–2.08)	1.18 (0.14–4.28)	4.89 (1.96–10.07)

of the Mode Selection Trial (MOST) with 312 patients showed that patients with one or more episodes of high atrial rates lasting more than 5 minutes had a 2.79-fold (CI, 1.51–5.15) increase in total mortality and stroke.[20] Patients with high atrial rate episodes were also more likely to develop longer episodes of AF later (hazard ratio 5.93; CI, 2.88–12.2). Another study correlating stroke risk in patients with a history of AF who were receiving devices showed that patients who had AF episodes greater than 1 day in duration after adjusting for other stroke risk factors had a hazard ratio of 3.1 (CI, 1.1–10.5).[21] These investigators did not find an increased risk of stroke in patients who had AF episodes more than 5 minutes, although they thought that it was due to 80% of their patient population having AF more than 5 minutes' duration, thus creating a lack of an appropriate comparison group.

Although the duration of AF seems important, it is also critical to combine considerations of AF burden with other risk factors. One study demonstrated that when using CHADS$_2$ score and AF burden in patients with pacemakers, patients with more than 24 hours of AF, and a CHADS$_2$ score of 1 had a risk of stroke of 5% compared with patients with a CHADS$_2$ score of 2 who were otherwise AF-free having a risk of stroke of 0.6%.[22] The highest risk of stroke (>5%) was seen in patients with CHADS2 of 3 or more regardless of their AF burden (**Fig. 1**).

Thus, although the exact amount of AF needed to incur an increased risk of stroke is unknown, it seems that even short episodes (<48 hours in duration) carry some risk.

Cryptogenic Stroke and Subclinical Atrial Fibrillation

Although the aforementioned studies suggest that evidence of subclinical AF picked up during routine monitoring performed for other reasons may identify a population at increased risk of thromboembolic events, another population to consider is those patients presenting with cryptogenic stroke. Subclinical AF can be a cause of ischemic stroke or transient ischemic attack but may often be difficult to pick up. Close to 15% of all strokes can be attributed directly to clinically known AF.[7,23–25] Up to 25% of patients, however, may have no identifiable cause of their stroke.[23,26,27] It is thought some of these cryptogenic strokes could be related to AF.[28] Various monitoring strategies have been used to pick up subclinical AF as a cause. Determining if AF is present in a patient with a prior stroke is important because anticoagulation can be initiated to reduce future risk or other changes in management may

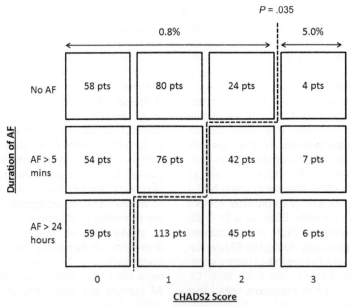

Fig. 1. Shown is the risk of thromboembolic events as a function of AF duration and CHADS$_2$ score. The figure demonstrates how the combination of CHADS$_2$ score and duration of AF episodes may discriminate the risk of thromboembolic events (*dashed line* separates the attendant risk). The number of patients (pts) in each group is listed in each box. Those at lower risk had an annual risk of 0.8% compared with 5% in the higher-risk group. (*Adapted from* Botto GL, Padeletti L, Santini M, et al. Presence and duration of atrial fibrillation detected by continuous monitoring: crucial implications for the risk of thromboembolic events. J Cardiovasc Electrophysiol 2009;20:241–8; with permission.)

occur.[29,30] The ideal choice of monitor, however, is unclear.

UTILITY OF SPECIFIC MONITORING MODALITIES IN DIAGNOSING AND MANAGING AF

The choice of a specific monitoring modality needs to take into consideration the duration over which monitoring is needed to establish a diagnosis, the reliance on symptoms to identify an episode of AF, and the burden to the patient. Types of monitoring include Holters, intermittent postevent monitors, TTMs, and ILRs. The potential utility of each in establishing a diagnosis of AF is discussed later.

Holter Monitoring

One retrospective review examined the utility of Holter monitoring in outpatients presenting for further work-up of a remote stroke.[31] Baseline ECG and Holter monitoring were done if thought necessary to try and establish a diagnosis of AF. There was a total of 200 patients included and only 3 (1.5%) patients had AF diagnosed by Holter in this series. Longer periods of Holter monitoring for up to 72 hours, however, have been shown beneficial.[32] In 82 patients with no prior history of AF, 72-hour Holter monitoring, obtained 2 to 3 weeks after a stroke, diagnosed AF in 5 (6%) patients, none of whom had symptoms during the AF event. AF was detected, however, in only 1 patient within 24 hours of initiating monitoring. Other patients had their first episode of AF between 24 and 48 hours (n = 2) or between 48 and 72 hours (n = 2). Another study examined even longer-term Holter monitoring for a course of 7 days.[33] AF was defined as an episode lasting more than 30 seconds. There were 24 patients (10%) who had AF detected. The study investigators also reported that patients found the Holter monitor cumbersome.

These data support the concept that longer-term monitoring may be necessary to accurately diagnose AF in the absence of a prior clinical history and that AF in these patients may often be subclinical. Most data, however, are in patients presenting with prior stroke or TIA and, thus, reflect an enriched population who may have a higher overall risk of AF. Whether these data may reflect the duration of monitoring needed to evaluate the efficacy of AF treatments, however, is unclear. If solely evaluating the efficacy of rate control, it is possible that a 24-hour Holter may be sufficient. When evaluating for the efficacy of rhythm control options, however, such as antiarrhythmic drugs or ablation, longer-term monitoring may be preferable.

Transtelephonic Monitoring and Monitored Telemetry

Long-term monitoring with monitored telemetry has been found more useful in diagnosing AF. In one study in which long-term (21-day) monitored telemetry was set up for 56 patients with cryptogenic stroke as outpatients postdischarge, AF was detected in 13 (23%) patients, with a median detection time of 7 days (range 2–19 days).[26] One caveat to broad screening of all patients, however, is cost. In the study, the cost of the monitoring using Medicare rates was $1124 per patient and $4841 per case of AF detected. Diagnosis of AF using this modality resulted in change of therapy in only 5 patients (antiplatelet medication changed to warfarin). Of the other patients, 6 (11%) were already maintained on warfarin, which they were taking before the stroke, and 2 (4%) patients were continued on antiplatelet medication alone. Thus, although there was apparent utility in diagnosing patients with AF, the impact on clinical management was not as clear from this study.

Another study of month-long TTMs in patients with a history of stroke and negative inpatient telemetry and Holter identified AF in as many as 9% of patients.[30] Only 2 of these patients had symptoms. Episodes ranged from 4 to 68 hours. The lower rate of detection with TTM than monitored telemetry may lie in the need for the patient to transmit data rather than having the rhythm continuously followed, as with monitored telemetry. With TTMs, however, there is still an improved likelihood of identifying AF compared with short-term Holter alone.

There is an ongoing trial examining the role of ILRs in patients with cryptogenic stroke.[34] The Cryptogenic Stroke and Underlying Atrial Fibrillation (CRYSTAL AF) trial is randomizing patients to either ILR or standard monitoring to see how it affects outcome. Trial results are expected to be available soon and these may guide clinicians better in choosing an appropriate monitoring strategy for detecting AF in this population. This trial may also assist in determining reasonable monitoring durations to accurately diagnose patients with AF. Currently, however, it seems that longer-term monitoring is better in diagnosing AF and the current data suggest that Holter monitoring yields the lowest (1.5% up to 6%) whereas TTM or monitored telemetry yields the highest (9%–27%) AF detection rates in this patient population.

REMOTE MONITORING FOR MANAGING PATIENTS WITH AF

The other area in which remote monitoring may prove beneficial is overall management of patients with previously diagnosed AF. This may range from evaluating the efficacy of rate control to evaluating for AF recurrence after ablation.

Monitoring Atrial Fibrillation Postablation

Radiofrequency catheter ablation has become an acceptable treatment of patients with symptomatic AF.[35–40] The AF ablation consensus document recommends that patients should be monitored postprocedure for 2 years using Holter (up to 7 days) or TTMs.[41] Patients who have had symptomatic AF also may have asymptomatic AF postablation and, therefore, such extended monitoring is needed to confirm that they are truly AF-free after the procedure. Prior studies have suggested that the incidence of asymptomatic AF in patients with paroxysmal AF may be as high as 4%.[42,43] In the setting of persistent AF after cardioversion, the rate of asymptomatic AF may be as high as 13%.[42] The utility of symptoms alone to monitor for recurrence in patients undergoing AF ablation may depend on the use of effective rate control, as suggested in one study using TTMs to monitor for AF late after ablation.[44]

Postablation monitoring with Holter versus TTM has been compared in prior studies.[45] In one study, patients (n = 72) who underwent catheter ablation for AF had both 24-hour Holter monitoring done at 30 and 120 days postablation and TTM initiated at 30 days postablation with daily transmissions for 90 days. With standard Holter monitoring and ECGs at 30 and 120 days, the incidence of AF recurrence was 13.9% compared with 27.8% for the TTM group (P<.01). Of those patients with recurrences, 10 had at least 1 asymptomatic episode and 8 were completely asymptomatic. Thus, in this population, extended monitoring with TTM doubled the recurrence rate compared with standard Holter monitoring.

It seems that longer-term monitoring postablation may identify more recurrences and alter management.[46] Kapa and colleagues[46] compared conventional monitoring (CM) with ILR in patients undergoing AF ablation. CM consisted of twice-daily 1-minute pulse rate assessment and 3 30-day TTM periods (at discharge 5 and 11 months) after the ablation. Over the 12-month study period, 13 patients (65%) in the ILR arm and 10 patients (56%) in the CM arm reported arrhythmia symptoms (P = .741). In only 3 patients in the ILR arm and 4 patients in the CM arm, however, did symptoms correlate with AF (total 7 of 23 patients [30%] reporting symptoms). In the remaining 16 patients (70%), the arrhythmia symptoms correlated with isolated atrial or ventricular premature beats or normal sinus rhythm. In the overall cohort, ILR

findings resulted in actionable events in 6 patients. In 5 patients, these events were marked bradycardia and/or asystole as a result of which 2 patients received pacemakers and 3 patients had antiarrhythmic drugs withdrawn. In 1 patient, ILR detected asymptomatic self-terminating ventricular tachycardia events, resulting in a change in medications. None of these events was detected by CM. The accuracy of ILR detection of AF was poor, however, with 915 episodes reported as AF, of which only 420 were adjudicated as true AF (accuracy = 46.0%). This differs from prior studies evaluating the utility of ILR in accurately identifying AF, although this may be due to differences in the method of adjudication of arrhythmia episodes.[47]

Utility of Postablation Monitoring

Postablation remote monitoring is important because it determines whether or not a patient may safely stop anticoagulation, may need a change in antiarrhythmic drugs, or may need a repeat ablation procedure. Symptoms are not always reliable discriminators of either the presence or absence of AF. Instead, there is a need for an objective measurement of the heart rhythm. In the first year, monitoring with an ILR can be beneficial. Monitoring may also provide reassurance to patients regarding AF cure when patients exhibit atypical symptoms because most symptoms do not reflect AF recurrence.

SUMMARY

Remote monitoring for AF is useful for many reasons. It can pick up asymptomatic AF, which can have important clinical consequences, including the need for long-term anticoagulation. In general, longer-term monitoring with TTM or monitored telemetry seems better in picking up AF than shorter-term Holter monitoring.

Cost of monitoring for longer periods of time always has to be taken into account. Increasing burden of AF has been associated with an increased risk of thromboembolic complications, although the exact burden of AF needed to prove benefit of initiating anticoagulant therapy remains unclear. Initiation of anticoagulation solely on the basis of short-lived bursts of AF can be a difficult choice.

Monitoring can also pick up incidental findings and change management in patients with already known AF. Specifically, monitoring may be useful in symptom-rhythm correlation. Evaluating the efficacy of therapies, such as ablation, also requires the use of monitoring. The choice of monitor (TTM or ILR), however, needs to take into account monitoring duration vis-à-vis ease and accuracy of arrhythmia detection.

Thus, the choice of monitoring modality needs to take into account several considerations. In turn, how to interpret and use the data need to be considered in the context of the available monitoring information. Future studies need to evaluate whether there may be a specific AF burden that may identify patients at higher risk of thromboembolic complications and whether there is a specific modality that may be ideal in the postablation management of patients with a history of AF.

REFERENCES

1. Lloyd-Jones D, Adams R, Carnethon M, et al. A report from the American Heart Association Statistics Committee and Stroke Statistics Subcommittee. Circulation 2009;119:e21–181.
2. Lloyd-Jones DM, Wang TJ, Leip EP, et al. Lifetime risk for development of atrial fibrillation: the Framingham Heart Study. Circulation 2004;110:1042–6.
3. Risk factors for stroke and efficacy of antithrombotic therapy in atrial fibrillation. Analysis of pooled data from five randomized controlled trials. Arch Intern Med 1994;154:1449–57.
4. Krahn AD, Manfreda J, Tate RB, et al. The natural history of atrial fibrillation: incidence, risk factors, and prognosis in the Manitoba Follow-Up Study. Am J Med 1995;98:476–84.
5. Dries DL, Exner DV, Gersh BJ, et al. Atrial fibrillation is associated with an increased risk for mortality and heart failure progression in patients with asymptomatic and symptomatic left ventricular systolic dysfunction: a retrospective analysis of the SOLVD trials. Studies of Left Ventricular Dysfunction. J Am Coll Cardiol 1998;32:695–703.
6. Benjamin EJ, Wolf PA, D'Agostino RB, et al. Impact of atrial fibrillation on the risk of death: the Framingham Heart Study. Circulation 1998;98:946–52.
7. Wolf PA, Abbott RD, Kannel WB. Atrial fibrillation as an independent risk factor for stroke: the Framingham Study. Stroke 1991;22:983–8.
8. Zimetbaum P, Goldman A. Ambulatory arrhythmia monitoring: choosing the right device. Circulation 2010;122:1629–36.
9. Gula LJ, Krahn AD, Massel D, et al. External loop recorders: determinants of diagnostic yield in patients with syncope. Am Heart J 2004;147:644–8.
10. Humphries KH, Kerr CR, Connolly SJ, et al. New-onset atrial fibrillation: sex differences in presentation, treatment, and outcome. Circulation 2001;103: 2365–70.
11. Kerr C, Boone J, Connolly S, et al. Follow-up of atrial fibrillation: the initial experience of the Canadian Registry of Atrial Fibrillation. Eur Heart J 1996; 17(Suppl C):48–51.
12. Kinlay S, Leitch JW, Neil A, et al. Cardiac event recorders yield more diagnoses and are more cost-effective than 48-hour Holter monitoring in patients with palpitations. A controlled clinical trial. Ann Intern Med 1996;124:16–20.
13. Page RL, Tilsch TW, Connolly SJ, et al. Asymptomatic or "silent" atrial fibrillation: frequency in untreated patients and patients receiving azimilide. Circulation 2003;107:1141–5.
14. Roche F, Gaspoz JM, Da Costa A, et al. Frequent and prolonged asymptomatic episodes of paroxysmal atrial fibrillation revealed by automatic long-term event recorders in patients with a negative 24-hour Holter. Pacing Clin Electrophysiol 2002;25: 1587–93.
15. Israel CW, Grönefeld G, Ehrlich JR, et al. Long-term risk of recurrent atrial fibrillation as documented by an implantable monitoring deviceImplications for optimal patient care. J Am Coll Cardiol 2004;43:47–52.
16. Wyse DG, Waldo AL, DiMarco JP, et al. A comparison of rate control and rhythm control in patients with atrial fibrillation. N Engl J Med 2002; 347:1825–33.
17. Van Gelder IC, Hagens VE, Bosker HA, et al. A comparison of rate control and rhythm control in patients with recurrent persistent atrial fibrillation. N Engl J Med 2002;347:1834–40.
18. Glotzer TV, Daoud EG, Wyse DG, et al. The relationship between daily atrial tachyarrhythmia burden from implantable device diagnostics and stroke risk: the TRENDS study. Circ Arrhythm Electrophysiol 2009;2:474–80.
19. Healey JS, Connolly SJ, Gold MR, et al. Subclinical atrial fibrillation and the risk of stroke. N Engl J Med 2012;366:120–9.
20. Glotzer TV, Hellkamp AS, Zimmerman J, et al. Atrial high rate episodes detected by pacemaker diagnostics predict death and stroke: report of the Atrial Diagnostics Ancillary Study of the MOde Selection Trial (MOST). Circulation 2003;107:1614–9.
21. Capucci A, Santini M, Padeletti L, et al. Monitored atrial fibrillation duration predicts arterial embolic events in patients suffering from bradycardia and atrial fibrillation implanted with antitachycardia pacemakers. J Am Coll Cardiol 2005;46:1913–20.
22. Botto GL, Padeletti L, Santini M, et al. Presence and duration of atrial fibrillation detected by continuous monitoring: crucial implications for the risk of thromboembolic events. J Cardiovasc Electrophysiol 2009;20:241–8.
23. Wolf PA, Dawber TR, Thomas HE Jr, et al. Epidemiologic assessment of chronic atrial fibrillation and risk of stroke: the Framingham study. Neurology 1978;28:973–7.
24. Wolf PA, Abbott RD, Kannel WB. Atrial fibrillation: a major contributor to stroke in the elderly. The Framingham Study. Arch Intern Med 1987;147:1561–4.

25. Petersen P, Godtfredsen J. Embolic complications in paroxysmal atrial fibrillation. Stroke 1986;17:622–6.
26. Tayal AH, Tian M, Kelly KM, et al. Atrial fibrillation detected by mobile cardiac outpatient telemetry in cryptogenic TIA or stroke. Neurology 2008;71: 1696–701.
27. Jabaudon D, Sztajzel J, Sievert K, et al. Usefulness of ambulatory 7-day ECG monitoring for the detection of atrial fibrillation and flutter after acute stroke and transient ischemic attack. Stroke 2004;35:1647–51.
28. Liao J, Khalid Z, Scallan C, et al. Noninvasive cardiac monitoring for detecting paroxysmal atrial fibrillation or flutter after acute ischemic stroke: a systematic review. Stroke 2007;38:2935–40.
29. Elijovich L, Josephson SA, Fung GL, et al. Intermittent atrial fibrillation may account for a large proportion of otherwise cryptogenic stroke: a study of 30-day cardiac event monitors. J Stroke Cerebrovasc Dis 2009;18:185–9.
30. Gaillard N, Deltour S, Vilotijevic B, et al. Detection of paroxysmal atrial fibrillation with transtelephonic EKG in TIA or stroke patients. Neurology 2010;74: 1666–70.
31. Douen A, Pageau N, Medic S. Usefulness of cardiovascular investigations in stroke management: clinical relevance and economic implications. Stroke 2007;38:1956–8.
32. Schuchert A, Behrens G, Meinertz T. Impact of long-term ECG recording on the detection of paroxysmal atrial fibrillation in patients after an acute ischemic stroke. Pacing Clin Electrophysiol 1999;22:1082–4.
33. Stahrenberg R, Weber-Kruger M, Seegers J, et al. Enhanced detection of paroxysmal atrial fibrillation by early and prolonged continuous holter monitoring in patients with cerebral ischemia presenting in sinus rhythm. Stroke 2010;41:2884–8.
34. Sinha AM, Diener HC, Morillo CA, et al. Cryptogenic Stroke and underlying Atrial Fibrillation (CRYSTAL AF): design and rationale. Am Heart J 2010;160: 36–41.e1.
35. Calkins H, Reynolds MR, Spector P, et al. Treatment of atrial fibrillation with antiarrhythmic drugs or radiofrequency ablation: two systematic literature reviews and meta-analyses. Circ Arrhythm Electrophysiol 2009;2:349–61.
36. Cappato R, Calkins H, Chen SA, et al. Updated worldwide survey on the methods, efficacy, and safety of catheter ablation for human atrial fibrillation. Circ Arrhythm Electrophysiol 2010;3:32–8.
37. Noheria A, Kumar A, Wylie JV Jr, et al. Catheter ablation vs antiarrhythmic drug therapy for atrial fibrillation: a systematic review. Arch Intern Med 2008;168:581–6.
38. Piccini JP, Lopes RD, Kong MH, et al. Pulmonary vein isolation for the maintenance of sinus rhythm in patients with atrial fibrillation: a meta-analysis of randomized, controlled trials. Circ Arrhythm Electrophysiol 2009;2:626–33.
39. Stabile G, Bertaglia E, Senatore G, et al. Catheter ablation treatment in patients with drug-refractory atrial fibrillation: a prospective, multi-centre, randomized, controlled study (Catheter Ablation for the Cure of Atrial Fibrillation Study). Eur Heart J 2006;27:216–21.
40. Terasawa T, Balk EM, Chung M, et al. Systematic review: comparative effectiveness of radiofrequency catheter ablation for atrial fibrillation. Ann Intern Med 2009;151:191–202.
41. Wann LS, Curtis AB, January CT, et al. 2011 ACCF/AHA/HRS focused update on the management of patients with atrial fibrillation (Updating the 2006 Guideline): a report of the American College of Cardiology Foundation/American Heart Association Task Force on Practice Guidelines. J Am Coll Cardiol 2011;57:223–42.
42. Page RL, Wilkinson WE, Clair WK, et al. Asymptomatic arrhythmias in patients with symptomatic paroxysmal atrial fibrillation and paroxysmal supraventricular tachycardia. Circulation 1994;89: 224–7.
43. Lin HJ, Wolf PA, Benjamin EJ, et al. Newly diagnosed atrial fibrillation and acute stroke. The Framingham Study. Stroke 1995;26:1527–30.
45. Oral H, Veerareddy S, Good E, et al. Prevalence of asymptomatic recurrences of atrial fibrillation after successful radiofrequency catheter ablation. J Cardiovasc Electrophysiol 2004;15:920–4.
44. Senatore G, Stabile G, Bertaglia E, et al. Role of transtelephonic electrocardiographic monitoring in detecting short-term arrhythmia recurrences after radiofrequency ablation in patients with atrial fibrillation. J Am Coll Cardiol 2005;45:873–6.
46. Kapa S, Epstein AE, Callans DJ, et al. Assessing arrhythmia burden after catheter ablation of atrial fibrillation using an implantable loop recorder: the ABACUS Study. J Cardiovasc Electrophysiol 2013. [Epub ahead of print].
47. Hindricks G, Pokushalov E, Urban L, et al. Performance of a new leadless implantable cardiac monitor in detecting and quantifying atrial fibrillation results of the XPECT trial. Circ Arrhythm Electrophysiol 2010;3:141–7.

State of the Art in Remote Monitoring Technology

K.L. Venkatachalam, MD[a], Samuel J. Asirvatham, MD[b],*

KEYWORDS

- Remote monitoring • Cardiac implantable electronic device • Cardiac monitoring • Telemedicine
- Mobile cardiac outpatient telemetry

KEY POINTS

- Remote monitoring of cardiac physiologic parameters, including heart rhythm and volume status, is playing an increasingly important role in the routine management of cardiac patients.
- This approach has the potential to provide significant cost and time savings to health care providers while reducing time for diagnosis and treatment of patients. It also has the ability to significantly enhance patient convenience by minimizing office visits.
- Integration of routine cardiac health parameters, such as blood pressure and daily weight, along with the possibility of monitoring serious changes, such as ST segment deviation, may make rapid, comprehensive cardiac care a reality in the near future.

INTRODUCTION

Although electronic and mechanical technologies to monitor cardiac status, such as sphygmomanometry and electrocardiography, have been available for approximately 150 years, true portability and ability to provide remote monitoring capabilities depended upon the invention of a viable electronic transistor in 1947. This development is considered by many technologists to be the most significant developments of the 20th century. Within a few years, reasonably priced commercial transistors made of germanium and silicon were available, and compact electronic amplifiers and analog signal processing circuit fabrication were feasible. The first practical, portable cardiac pacemaker, built in 1957, was based on a metronome circuit taken from an electronics magazine. The invention of the integrated circuit and the microprocessor represented a giant leap forward in the quest for compact, reliable electronic monitoring systems. Since then, portable rhythm monitoring using on-board storage, implantable defibrillators, pressure and volume sensors, and mobile cardiac telemetry have been developed, greatly improving the ease and rapidity of diagnosis and treatment. New applications of these technologies are revealed on a regular basis and well-done studies have demonstrated the usefulness of these technologies to caregivers and patients. Expert consensus statements have also been developed to guide clinicians on the use of these technologies.[1]

TECHNOLOGY

The heart of any cardiac electronic monitoring system is the sensor and its associated electronic circuitry. The simplest sensors for monitoring cardiac electrical activity consist of tabs of silver-silver chloride with a conductive gel to reduce skin impedance. These can be used to transduce heart rate as well as rhythm and morphology. Polymer versions of these electrodes have also been

Disclosures: The authors have nothing to disclose.
[a] Department of Medicine, Division of Cardiology, Mayo Clinic Florida, 4500 San Pablo Road, Davis 7, Jacksonville, FL 32224, USA; [b] Department of Medicine, Division of Cardiology, Saint Mary's Hospital, Mayo Clinic Minnesota, Mary Brigh Building 4-523, 1216 2nd Street Southwest, Rochester, MN 55902, USA
* Corresponding author.
E-mail address: asirvatham.samuel@mayo.edu

Card Electrophysiol Clin 5 (2013) 365–370
http://dx.doi.org/10.1016/j.ccep.2013.05.001
1877-9182/13/$ – see front matter © 2013 Elsevier Inc. All rights reserved.

developed with adhesive backing and are also available in hypoallergenic versions, which can be extremely helpful during long-term monitoring in patients with sensitive skin. These same electrodes may be used to monitor respiration by injecting small, high-frequency currents through the chest and measuring impedance changes, which correlate with respiration rate. Small piezoelectric crystals can also be used as motion sensors to detect patient activity level and can correlate activity with rhythm, a useful diagnostic tool. All of these features may be integrated into a single, composite, easy-to-apply sensor package. A recent example of such a commercial device is the BodyGuardian Remote Monitoring System (Preventice, Minneapolis, Minnesota).

Microelectromechanical systems (MEMS) technology has produced a remarkable array of silicon, polymer, ceramic, and metal transducers, which can measure acceleration (activity) as well as pressure in cardiac monitors. These devices can be fabricated using lithography and etching techniques originally developed for semiconductor manufacturing and can be made exceedingly small. Bulk manufacturing also allows for inexpensive precalibrated transducers that can be used in noninvasive and invasive applications.[2]

Miniature thermistors (resistors whose resistance decreases in predictable fashion with increasing temperature) and thermocouples (metal alloy junctions whose voltage changes predictably with changes in temperature) are used routinely for temperature sensing in a variety of medical applications also.

Injecting small, high-frequency currents through external chest electrodes or internal defibrillator electrodes can provide additional useful information on pulmonary congestion by monitoring changes in absolute impedance. This technique has allowed for early warning in the recognition and treatment of heart failure exacerbation, confirmed by clinical studies.[3,4]

The outputs of these sensors (voltage, current, and impedance) need to be amplified, filtered, and processed before they can be interpreted to provide useful information. The basic building block for signal processing is the electronic instrumentation amplifier, which provides high levels of amplification (signal increase) while rejecting noise (unwanted signals) to a significant degree. The amplified signal is then filtered, initially using hardware-based filters to limit noise and motion artifact. The amplified, filtered signal is then digitized with an analog-to-digital converter.[5] The digital data may then be stored, manipulated, or transmitted using a variety of techniques (**Fig. 1**). Memory cost and density have improved

dramatically over the past 20 years, allowing for storage of significant amounts of high-quality physiologic data locally on a medical device.

The data may be transmitted back to the clinical facility using radiofrequency energy from a patient's device, manually or automatically, using the Industrial, Scientific, and Medical band or the cellular Global System for Mobile Communications bands. The received data are then subjected to more powerful digital signal processing techniques to clean up the signals and extract small signals from noise to allow accurate measurement. The measured data are then displayed either graphically or in tabular form for medical interpretation.

Increased understanding of cardiac physiology coupled with the evolution of electronic and medical technology has produced a useful set of tools to remotely monitor important cardiac parameters and deliver that information to appropriate clinical staff for prompt follow-up.

STATE OF THE ART IN REMOTE CARDIAC PARAMETER MONITORING

Remote cardiac monitoring may be divided into several areas: rhythm monitoring for diagnostic purposes, pressure and volume monitoring to assess heart failure status, lead and device integrity monitoring, and monitoring efficacy of therapies, such as ablation procedures for dysrhythmias.

Rhythm Monitoring

Rhythm monitoring for diagnosis of palpitations, near-syncope, and syncope is excellent for correlating symptoms and rhythms in the nonmedical setting; 24-hour Holter monitors can provide information on heart rate range and averages, assess for chronotropic incompetence, and inform on arrhythmia burden, also allowing monitoring of treatment efficacy. Although the monitoring itself is remote to the medical facility, the data are stored on board the device and may be downloaded after the required duration. Event monitors allow patients to document symptoms and monitor rhythms for up to 4 weeks, with periodic downloads performed by the patient through a telephone connection. Multilead event monitors, such as the Intelli-Heart monitor (Intelli-Heart Services, Los Angeles, California) can also measure QT intervals beat-by-beat for extended periods to assess for dynamic lengthening of QT intervals in suspected long-QT syndromes. Periodic monitoring with such devices is also used routinely by clinicians to assess efficacy of therapeutic procedures, such as atrial fibrillation ablation, to determine if

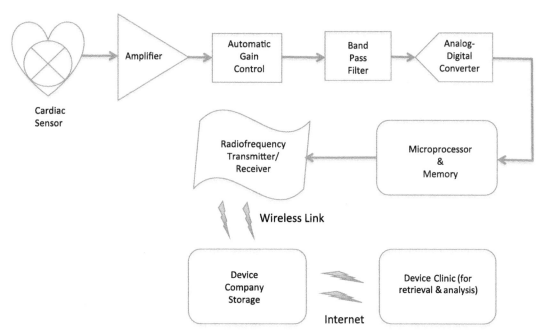

Fig. 1. Block diagram representing a typical cardiac remote monitoring system. The cardiac sensor's output (voltage, current, pressure, and impedance) is amplified. The amplitude may be adjusted dynamically by the system using an automatic gain control circuit before band-pass filtering the signal. It is converted from analog data to digital information by the analog-digital converter. The digital data are transmitted using radiofrequency energy to the data storage system of the device manufacturer. These data are available to qualified health care personnel in device clinics via download using an Internet connection. They can then communicate via telephone to the patient regarding symptoms and therapy.

patients are candidates for discontinuation of anti-coagulation. Mobile cardiac outpatient telemetry devices can continuously transmit rhythm data from patients by wireless communication to a central monitoring station, where trained personnel analyze and categorize rhythm abnormalities in real time, alerting the appropriate clinical staff at the ordering facility of any serious arrhythmias, such as ventricular tachycardia or prolonged sinus pauses.

Patient acceptance of external patches and the bulk of the attached electronic devices usually limit the use of such products to a few weeks of monitoring. In cases where symptomatic episodes are infrequent (eg, syncopal spells every few months), implantable loop recorders have demonstrated their usefulness unequivocally.[6] These leadless devices, implanted with a quick and simple surgical procedure in the left chest wall, can remain implanted for more than 3 years and provide valuable information on symptom/rhythm correlation. Such devices are also increasingly used for diagnosing atrial fibrillation as the cause of some cases of cryptogenic stroke. An ongoing Spanish trial, CRYPTONITE, will be completed in 2013.

Heart Failure Monitoring

Patient volume status and assessment of intra-cardiac pressures remotely have received intense scrutiny from heart failure specialists over the past several years. Approximately 1 million heart failure hospitalizations occur in the United States annually, with a 30-day readmission rate of 27%,[7] placing an enormous burden on health care resources. Several early trials, including Telemonitoring to Improve Heart Failure Outcomes[8] and Telemedical Interventional Monitoring in Heart Failure,[9] were not able to demonstrate a positive impact of telemonitoring on heart failure–related rehospitalizations or mortality. Dedicated intra-cardiac pressure monitors, such as the right ventricular pressure sensor in the Chronicle device (Medtronic, Minneapolis, Minnesota) and the left atrial pressure sensor in HeartPOD (St. Jude Medical, Minneapolis, Minnesota), provide indirect or direct assessment of left ventricular filling pressures. The initial results of the Chronicle Offers Management to Patients with Advanced Signs and Symptoms of Heart Failure trial, which used the Chronicle device, did not find a significant difference in heart failure events between the intervention and control groups. Subsequent analysis suggested, however, that persistently high filling pressures recorded by Chronicle, irrespective of symptoms, placed people at higher risk for hospitalization.[10] An observational study, Hemodynamically Guided Home Self-Therapy in Severe Heart Failure Patients (HOMEOSTASIS), in New York Heart Association Class III and Class IV patients, using the HeartPOD, had a lower risk of acute decompensation or death.[11] Accurate measurement of pulmonary artery pressure using a MEMS sensor implanted in the pulmonary artery showed a 30% reduction in heart failure hospitalizations in New York Heart Association Class III patients.[12] This study (CHAMPION [CardioMEMS Heart Sensor Allows Monitoring of Pressure to Improve Outcomes in NYHA Class III Patients]) also showed that a comprehensive approach to patient management using the pressure data, with guidelines on medication adjustment provided to clinicians, improved the chance of good outcomes in these patients. OptiVol (Medtronic, Minneapolis, Minnesota) technology measures heart failure exacerbation by monitoring changes in lung impedance, which can alert clinicians to impending episodes of heart failure, prompting early treatment.[13]

Heart failure management systems have also been developed (Latitude, Boston Scientific, St. Paul, Minnesota) that integrate daily weight measurement with daily blood pressure and symptom self-reports. The digital outputs of each of the separate devices that make up this system connect to the Latitude communicator via a short-range radiofrequency communication system (Bluetooth), and the composite data can be retrieved by a patient's clinician to evaluate treatment efficacy and assess for impending heart failure exacerbation.

Device and Lead Integrity Monitoring

Despite the exceedingly stringent working environment of pacemaker and defibrillator leads (100,000 flexions per day for 20–30 years), device manufacturers have developed reliable systems overall. There have been a few instances, however, of lead failures and lead integrity problems that have led to advisories as well as lead recalls, with a significant burden on patients and clinicians. Algorithms to monitor lead integrity remotely have now been incorporated into the device software of most implanted cardiac devices, with the ability to alert patients as well as physicians about potential lead problems triggered by excessive noise, significant impedance changes, or large changes in sensed voltages. The implications of all of these data sent by patients manually and automatically to pacemaker

clinics can be huge. Transmissions not requiring any action may be processed rapidly but clinically important transmissions can dramatically increase the workload on any given day in a clinic.[14,15]

MONITORING EFFICACY OF THERAPY

Monitoring patients for extended periods after ablation for atrial fibrillation is a promising new area for use of remote monitors, which could be exceptionally useful in determining long-term efficacy of various ablation procedures, the need for long-term anticoagulation in selected patients, and correlation between nonatrial fibrillation-related symptoms and rhythms. Patients with preexisting dual-chamber pacemakers or defibrillators can continue routine monitoring of their devices and evaluation of atrial high rate episodes, which may point to atrial flutter or atrial fibrillation recurrence. An alternative, not currently reimbursed, is to implant a loop recorder for 3 years of data. A noninvasive approach involves external cardiac monitors placed every few months for 7 to 10 days to sample patient rhythms to detect silent episodes of atrial fibrillation.

Manufacturers of all implanted defibrillators and some implantable pacemakers offer wireless remote monitoring. Routine device parameters measured include battery status, lead integrity checks, capture and sensing, and arrhythmia episodes. The data are automatically retrieved from the device by a home monitor that then transmits the information via a telephone connection (wired or mobile) to the manufacturer's servers. The data can then be downloaded via the Internet by individual pacemaker clinic staff and displayed on commercial software such as Paceart (Medtronic, Minneapolis, Minnesota). Patients may also activate a download based on symptoms, with requested callbacks from the appropriate pacemaker clinic. This has definitely improved patient convenience although there has also been some resistance to the use of this technology by patients. Simplification of the communication process (technology) and the realization that this is an effective way to monitor their devices should increase patient compliance.

THE FUTURE

Remote cardiac monitoring has entered an exciting phase in its development, with rapid technologic advance supported by increasing clinician and patient awareness and acceptance. As more wireless bandwidth becomes available to the medical community, more useful data can be downloaded quickly, improving perceived convenience. Smartphone applications have already been developed to allow patients to monitor pulse rate (with no additional hardware) or record rhythms (with small data acquisition hardware attachments) and transmit the information to their clinicians for rapid response to symptoms. This increases the burden on clinicians, and mechanisms to handle the significant increase in clinical data need to be developed before it becomes overwhelming. Compact hardware solutions to improve the reliability of rate and rhythm monitoring with sophisticated software algorithms providing immediate diagnoses with reasonable accuracy are being developed and will be available to general cardiac health care consumers in the near future. An exciting addition to this development is the possibility of monitoring ST segment deviations associated with cardiac ischemia in high-risk patients.[16] This was tested in 2 pilot studies (DETECT and Cardiosaver) in 37 patients with an implanted device, the AngelMed Guardian implantable ischemia detection system (Angel Medical Systems, Shrewsbury, New Jersey), designed to measure ST segment deviations on a beat-by-beat basis and compare them to a moving average. Over a mean follow-up of 1.5 years, 4 patients had ST segment shifts (7 events) related to heart rate changes, prompting an alarm from the device, urging the patients to be evaluated at a local emergency department for true supply-related ischemic events. The mean alarm-to-door time was 26.5 minutes, substantially less than the 144 minutes observed in the general ST elevation myocardial infarction population. This technology, when improved to minimize false alarms, has the potential to significantly reduce time-to-treatment in high-risk cardiac patients and could be incorporated into standard implantable defibrillator designs in the not-too-distant future.

Overall, the future looks bright for cardiac remote monitoring. Confirming that such technology, when used appropriately for patient management, can reduce health care costs in the long run will also provide the impetus for reasonable financial reimbursement. Clinicians deluged with the anticipated data from all this remote cardiac monitoring will have to work out approaches to provide smooth workflow in device clinics to minimize frustration in patients and health care staff while efficiently handling the true clinical emergencies revealed by the monitoring.

REFERENCES

1. Dubner S, Auricchio A, Steinberg JS, et al. ISHNE/EHRA expert consensus on remote monitoring of cardiovascular implantable electronic devices (CIEDs). Europace 2012;14:278–93.

2. Anand IS, Greenberg BH, Fogoros RN, et al. Design of the multi-sensor monitoring in congestive heart failure (music) study: prospective trial to assess the utility of continuous wireless physiologic monitoring in heart failure. J Card Fail 2011;17:11–6.

3. Bui AL, Fonarow GC. Home monitoring for heart failure management. J Am Coll Cardiol 2012;59:97–104.

4. Anand IS, Tang WH, Greenberg BH, et al. Design and performance of a multisensor heart failure monitoring algorithm: results from the multisensor monitoring in congestive heart failure (music) study. J Card Fail 2012;18:289–95.

5. Venkatachalam KL, Herbrandson JE, Asirvatham SJ. Signals and signal processing for the electrophysiologist: part ii: signal processing and artifact. Circ Arrhythm Electrophysiol 2011;4:974–81.

6. Krahn AD, Klein GJ, Skanes AC, et al. Use of the implantable loop recorder in evaluation of patients with unexplained syncope. J Cardiovasc Electrophysiol 2003;14:S70–3.

7. Jencks SF, Williams MV, Coleman EA. Rehospitalizations among patients in the medicare fee-for-service program. N Engl J Med 2009;360:1418–28.

8. Chaudhry SI, Mattera JA, Curtis JP, et al. Telemonitoring in patients with heart failure. N Engl J Med 2010;363:2301–9.

9. Koehler F, Winkler S, Schieber M, et al. Impact of remote telemedical management on mortality and hospitalizations in ambulatory patients with chronic heart failure: the telemedical interventional monitoring in heart failure study. Circulation 2011;123:1873–80.

10. Stevenson LW, Zile M, Bennett TD, et al. Chronic ambulatory intracardiac pressures and future heart failure events. Circ Heart Fail 2010;3:580–7.

11. Ritzema J, Troughton R, Melton I, et al. Physician-directed patient self-management of left atrial pressure in advanced chronic heart failure. Circulation 2010;121:1086–95.

12. Abraham WT, Adamson PB, Bourge RC, et al. Wireless pulmonary artery haemodynamic monitoring in chronic heart failure: a randomised controlled trial. Lancet 2011;377:658–66.

13. Varma N, Michalski J, Epstein AE, et al. Automatic remote monitoring of implantable cardioverter-defibrillator lead and generator performance: the lumos-t safely reduces routine office device follow-up (trust) trial. Circ Arrhythm Electrophysiol 2010;3:428–36.

14. Cronin EM, Ching EA, Varma N, et al. Remote monitoring of cardiovascular devices: a time and activity analysis. Heart Rhythm 2012;9:1947–51.

15. Landolina M, Perego GB, Lunati M, et al. Remote monitoring reduces healthcare use and improves

quality of care in heart failure patients with implantable defibrillators: the evolution of management strategies of heart failure patients with implantable defibrillators (evolvo) study. Circulation 2012;125: 2985–92.

16. Fischell TA, Fischell DR, Avezum A, et al. Initial clinical results using intracardiac electrogram monitoring to detect and alert patients during coronary plaque rupture and ischemia. J Am Coll Cardiol 2010;56:1089–98.

Future Trends in the Evolution of Remote Monitoring and Physiologic Sensing Technologies

Suraj Kapa, MD[a], Jonathan P. Man, MD[b],
Gregory E. Supple, MD[b],*

KEYWORDS

• Remote monitoring • Physiologic sensors • Heart failure • Arrhythmia

KEY POINTS

• Clinical use of remote monitoring is trending toward greater use of wireless transmission, which is less dependent on the patient transmitting their own data.
• Advances in wireless transmission, smaller technologies, and applications on smartphones may allow for the easier monitoring of patients in the ambulatory setting.
• Advances in physiologic sensors for heart failure, blood pressure, and other biological parameters may improve management of patients in the long-term but still requires research as to clinical validity and efficacy.
• Future technologies will require extensive validation, especially in terms of data management and evaluation of cost-effectiveness.

INTRODUCTION

Monitoring technologies have evolved significantly over the course of the past several decades, from Holter monitors, which require patients to wear leads continuously over the course of days and physically return the monitors, to modern Wi-Fi–equipped implantable devices, which cause minimal encumbrance to the patient. Most cardiac monitoring equipment focuses on the recording and assessment of heart rhythm and, in turn, on correlating abnormal rhythms with symptoms. More modern-day devices have taken this a step further and include pressure and impedance monitors to evaluate physiologic parameters ranging from intracardiac pressure to pulmonary edema in the setting of heart failure. However, data are still lacking on their usefulness, and technology continues to improve.

With the rapid evolution and miniaturization of computing technology in addition to development of better biocompatible materials, the potential for future monitors and physiologic sensors is vast. Future devices may invoke already existing technology that may be integrated in unique ways. These developments will be critical to improvements in the ambulatory care of patients, especially as trends in health care push more toward favoring outpatient over inpatient care.[1,2] The ability to closely monitor and manage patients at home may offer the ability to change the face of day-to-day patient care. However, this evolution

Disclosures: The authors have nothing to disclose.
[a] Division of Cardiology, Mayo Clinic College of Medicine, 200 First Street SW, Rochester, MN 55905, USA;
[b] Division of Cardiac Electrophysiology, Department of Medicine, University of Pennsylvania, 3400 Spruce Street, Philadelphia, PA 19104, USA
* Corresponding author.
E-mail address: Gregory.supple@uphs.upenn.edu

will depend on the development of novel technologies, validation of their clinical accuracy and benefit, and evaluation of their cost.[3]

This review pinpoints potential future trends in the development of remote monitoring technology. It also focuses on physiologic sensing technologies and how physiologic sensors may be integrated into existing technology or be developed as stand-alone technologies for the purposes of patient care.

GENERAL TRENDS IN REMOTE MONITORING

Monitoring methods may be widely separated into invasive and noninvasive methods. Invasive technologies generally require a surgical incision, with placement of an implantable device either subcutaneously or submuscularly, with or without intravascular wires. Noninvasive monitors typically consist of externally placed stickers, which can detect the heart rhythm, and an externally worn device. Invasive methods stop patients from worrying about making sure that the electrocardiographic stickers stay attached (eg, in the shower) and minimize encumbrance in terms of daily activities. However, many patients may still find implantable monitors unsatisfactory, because they require a small incision, and some patients may experience discomfort related to the device.[4] In turn, noninvasive methods are often cumbersome and generally depend on the patient to physically transmit data. Most noninvasive monitoring technologies function to evaluate only heart rate and rhythm and not other physiologic parameters. The same is true of invasive devices, although some modern pacemakers and defibrillators can evaluate heart failure status via indirect methods. Some home monitoring systems for pacemakers and defibrillators also allow the patient to transmit their blood pressure and daily weight along with device data.

The overall trend for monitoring technologies has consisted of both making smaller, less cumbersome devices as well as offering real-time assessments that depend less and less on the patient transmitting their own data. The wide availability of cellular networks, Wi-Fi, Bluetooth, and other wireless systems has allowed for more rapid transmission of data directly from devices to central databases.[5,6] However, many technologies still rely on a landline to transmit data over a network.

In turn, devices are also becoming smaller and less reliant on patient interaction with the device for the placement and removal of stickers or the monitor itself. For example, a new external monitor (Zio Patch, iRhythm, San Francisco, CA) may be placed on the body, stay in place for up to 14 days, and is not affected by exposure to water or other elements. Advances such as these may make noninvasive electrocardiographic monitors more appealing to patients and, in turn, improve compliance.[7] Data suggest that the usefulness of noninvasive monitors in identifying arrhythmias lies largely in the duration of monitoring, which in turn involves the patient wearing or using the monitor over the intended period.[8–10]

SMARTPHONES IN OUTPATIENT MONITORING

Advances in cellular technology have allowed for the development of a wide array of applications for smartphones. Use of these phones, which are often continuously connected to both a cellular and data network, may allow patients to easily track their own data day to day and transmit these data.[11,12] Several recent applications have invoked ways of using existing cellular technology to record the heart rhythm and determine everything from heart rate to the regularity of the rhythm, which may assist patients in determining when they are in atrial fibrillation or for symptom-rhythm correlation. Studies of use of these applications have suggested that a recorded irregular pulse may accurately and cost-effectively identify patients with frequent premature atrial or ventricular contractions or atrial fibrillation (**Fig. 1**).[13]

However, the potential use of smartphones for home monitoring may extend beyond the monitoring of heart rhythm alone. Applications including urine screening for markers of a variety of diseases and methods of tracking daily physical activity have been developed.[14–17] The ability to identify diseases early in their course (especially for patients who are not close to a physician's office or hospital) or to evaluate the activity level of a patient may allow physicians to more quickly or effectively discuss changes in clinical management with patients.

Although these smartphone applications have evolved rapidly, there are several important caveats. First, as with any medical test, validation of the data obtained via these applications needs to be performed. Wide availability of self-testing for disease processes may also increase health care costs if patients with a low pretest probability of disease seek physician evaluation because of abnormal tests that do not otherwise have any clinical significance.

Another important consideration is liability. When data are obtained that may suggest the presence of an abnormality, who is responsible

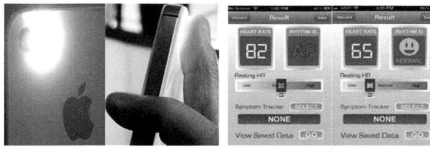

Fig. 1. Example of an application used to evaluate for atrial fibrillation using a smartphone. From left to right, the first panel shows the iPhone 4S (Apple Inc., Cupertino, CA) camera, the second panel shows the finger applied to the camera such that it can detect the pulse, the third panel shows a screenshot of the application when a patient is in atrial fibrillation, and the last panel shows a screenshot of the application when a patient is in sinus rhythm. (*From* McManus DD, Lee J, Maitas O, et al. A novel application for the detection of an irregular pulse using an iPhone 4S in patients with atrial fibrillation. Heart Rhythm 2013;10:316; with permission.)

for acting on the information obtained? For example, if a patient uses a smartphone application to track their heart rate or rhythm and calls their physician to report arrhythmia recurrence based on the smartphone application, which subsequently results in a change in medication, who is responsible if the primary data were wrong? This situation raises the critical importance of both validating the software that is developed and having systems in place to define certain applications as health care grade, or of sufficient quality that they may be used to acquire data for routine clinical management of patients.

DEDICATED WIRELESS NETWORKS

Manufacturers of implantable devices are increasingly relying on wireless data transmission to the point that patients may simply walk by a central terminal placed in their home that can automatically communicate with the device and store and transmit data. However, many modern monitoring technologies including both implantable and noninvasive devices still use landlines. As the cost of wireless network use decreases and availability is more widespread, more devices will likely adopt similar means of transmission, allowing for more real-time and seamless transmission of data to a central network and to the clinician.

However, one of the considerations in the evolution of such technology lies in the availability of wireless access points in remote areas and the impact of potential data overload on clinicians.[18] First, rural locations do not necessarily have the same access to cellular and wireless networks. Thus, traditional methods such as office visits, landlines for data transmission, and delivery of external monitors by mail will continue to be necessary. Second, daily transmissions of data

need to be reviewed on a continuous basis, and mechanisms for managing these data are necessary.[19,20] For certain monitoring systems, such as transtelephonic monitors or monitored telemetry, a technician can access and review the transmissions and decide when to inform the clinician of an important finding. However, such a service is usually not available for implantable devices and depends on the clinician finding a way to parse through the data. Often, there is a high rate of inappropriate diagnosis with algorithms used by implantable devices to identify arrhythmias, and, thus, clinician review of tracings is important to ensure accuracy. If the patient has a high frequency of incidental findings (eg, asymptomatic bradyarrhythmias or asymptomatic paroxysmal atrial fibrillation), this can create excessive data for the clinician to deal with.

However, the use of wireless transmissions that can automatically send information from devices to the clinician holds many potential future benefits in the diagnosis and care of patients, including early identification of devices reaching end of life, of arrhythmia occurrence, or of disease progression, such as with hypertension.[21,22]

IMPLANTABLE LOOP RECORDERS

Implantable loop recorders are useful as a minimally invasive tool to monitor the heart rhythm. Current devices are approximately the size of a USB (Universal Serial Bus) drive and can be used for up to 3 years to continuously monitor the heart rhythm. Multiple studies have suggested usefulness in evaluating for arrhythmias in patients with rare symptoms that may not be otherwise identified by traditional noninvasive monitors (**Fig. 2**).[4,23,24] Implantation requires a sterile environment and creation of a small incision. Their value lies in the

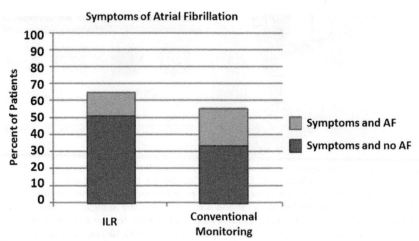

Fig. 2. Percentage of patients with an implantable loop recorder (ILR) and conventional monitoring who reported symptoms suggestive of arrhythmia recurrence cross-checked for accuracy via ILR over a 12-month study period. Only in a few patients did symptoms correlate with true arrhythmia recurrence. AF, atrial fibrillation. (*From* Kapa S, Epstein AE, Callans DJ, et al. Assessing arrhythmia burden after catheter ablation of atrial fibrillation using an implantable loop recorder: The ABACUS Study. J Cardiovasc Electrophysiol 2013. [Epub ahead of print], http://dx.doi.org/10.1111/jce.12141; with permission.)

multiple limitations including patient compliance with wearable monitor systems.[25]

The issue with current loop recorders still includes their size, the need for a sterile environment (in most institutions, an operating room), and the algorithms used for arrhythmia detection. Future devices under development are aimed at further miniaturization, to the point that they can be implanted at the bedside or in the ambulatory setting. These devices would be about the size of a pin. However, the main hurdle is in developing accurate algorithms for arrhythmia detection. Just as with other implantable devices, the loop recorder is only as good as the programming used to detect arrhythmias. Limitations in the algorithms may make detection of certain arrhythmias, such as atrial fibrillation, fraught with difficulty because of the high rate of false-positive results.[4,26] Review of every tracing by a clinician may be arduous depending on the total number of episodes recorded. Thus, improvements in the algorithms or identifying how to best tailor algorithms to patient needs will be required to identify the way to most effectively use these devices.

MONITORING OF THE ELECTROCARDIOGRAM BEYOND THE RATE AND RHYTHM

Current technology is relatively effective at monitoring changes in heart rate and rhythm. Most cardiac monitoring is aimed at these 2 patient parameters. However, electrocardiographic monitoring holds the potential for clinical evaluation

beyond the rate and rhythm.[27] For example, in patients on antiarrhythmic medications that prolong the QT interval, it may be possible to continuously evaluate the QT interval in the ambulatory setting.[28,29] Although medications such as dofetilide or sotalol are generally loaded in the inpatient setting, it is still possible that changes in diet or other medications may affect drug metabolism, which can, in turn, affect the QT interval after the patient returns home. In turn, electrolyte abnormalities caused by illness or another cause may similarly affect the drug effect on the QT interval. Thus, in patients with certain types of monitors, such as loop recorders or noninvasive monitors, algorithms to monitor the QT interval may be possible.

THE FUTURE OF PHYSIOLOGIC SENSING

Modern-day pacemakers and defibrillators may use pressure or impedance sensors to evaluate for volume or pressure overload in the setting of heart failure. The data on these sensors in terms of accuracy and usefulness have been mixed, although they suggest improved event-free survival and decreased hospitalizations.[30–32] These sensors provide an initial example of how implantable devices may afford a way to monitor a variety of cardiovascular parameters beyond just heart rate and rhythm. However, one of the limitations of any physiologic sensor is in identifying an indication for implantation as a stand-alone technology as opposed to as an adjunct to a device being implanted for other reasons (such as a pacemaker or defibrillator).

Heart Failure Monitoring

The goal of invasive monitors to evaluate heart failure status is to attempt to prevent hospitalizations by allowing clinicians to intervene in the ambulatory setting before patients reach a more advanced level of decompensation, which would not be treatable with oral medications alone.[30–32] The oldest means of remote monitoring involved patients recording their own body weight, heart rate, blood pressure, and other parameters and then relaying this information to the physician either on a regular basis or when certain set points were exceeded (eg, a weight gain beyond a previously discussed amount). More modern implantable devices have been used to invasively monitor parameters such as heart rate variability, physical activity level through use of accelerometers, pressure sensors, impedance monitoring, or Doppler recording of cardiac output.

One trend in the use of these invasive monitors has been developing new algorithms that use more than 1 sensor.[30,33] However, the best combination of sensors is unclear. Furthermore, whether such sensors should provide an alert to the patient as opposed to the clinician, especially in situations in which patients are not transmitting device data regularly, is unclear.

Future sensing technology in heart failure may use biomarker detection as well.[30,34–36] Detecting biomarker levels in blood flowing past intravascular catheters may allow for detection of natriuretic peptides or inflammatory markers that correlate with heart failure status. In turn, these biomarker levels can be used, similar to information obtained from impedance or pressure sensors, to detect when patients require changes in their heart failure therapy.

Blood Pressure Monitoring

There have been recent advances in invasive blood pressure monitors that can track blood pressure over long periods.[22,37–39] One example is a device that can be implanted via a small incision and wrapped around a small blood vessel for continuous recording of arterial pressure (**Fig. 3**).[40] The use of biocompatible materials has made the development of these devices possible. However, depending on the vessel used, the pressure sensed may be reflective of central versus peripheral pressure, and studies are needed to identify where and how best to implant such devices. Furthermore, how such monitors would be used in clinical practice needs to be evaluated. One way in which these monitors can be beneficial is to more accurately monitor the effect of blood pressure therapies at home rather than relying on home sphygmomanometers, which depend on the patient checking their own pressure and proper calibration. Risk, benefit, and cost-effectiveness of the more accurate and intensive and invasive blood pressure monitoring in the treatment of hypertension would have to be carefully studied.

Biomarker Tracking and Drug Assays

Two areas in which future technologies may help in the care of the cardiac patient include the ability to track biomarkers and drug levels. Although implantable monitors have been studied for glucose monitoring, there is theoretic potential for

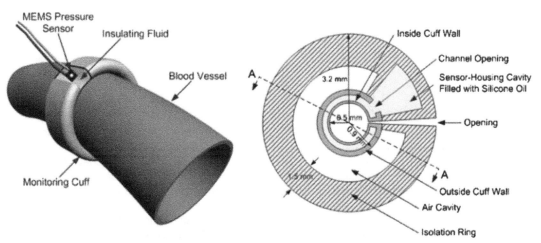

Fig. 3. Example of an implantable blood pressure monitor described by Cong and colleagues.[40] MEMS, microelectromechanical systems. (*From* Potkay JA. Long term, implantable blood pressure monitoring systems. Biomed Microdevices 2008;10:388; with permission.)

extending monitoring to other biomarkers.[41,42] Biomarkers relevant to the electrophysiology patient may include heart failure markers as noted earlier or troponin levels, especially in patients with coronary disease. Sudden changes in troponin may alert the patient and the clinician to concern for an acute coronary event. Or, in turn, acute coronary syndrome may be more rapidly ruled out in combination with traditional hospital-based assays.

Tracking of anticoagulation is another example of potential advancement in sensing technologies. Tracking the international normalized ratio via the implanted device as opposed to using a home monitoring system that would require fingersticks may offer additional benefit by allowing for a more automated system. An alert system may be used for an excessive decrease or increase in the level of anticoagulation. However, again, such systems would require extensive validation, and the use of such a technology at this stage may be relevant only in patients who already have implantable devices for other reasons.

Monitoring of drug levels at home may also be useful in certain patients. For example, it may be possible to use an assay to evaluate digoxin or other drug levels. This assay may be particularly useful with medications that have a narrow therapeutic range. Such assays may also allow clinicians to better assess drug compliance.

Drug Delivery Systems

One potential advance that would make implantation of physiologic sensors useful is if there was a mechanism for the device to deliver a pharmacologic or other therapy in response to physiologic perturbations.[43,44] For example, if there was a system for a device to detect the level of anticoagulation and suggest alterations in anticoagulant dosing, or for a device to deliver a drug directly (such as an antiarrhythmic drug in response to a change in rhythm or a rate control agent after accounting for level of activity and heart rate), this could offer a closed loop wherein diagnosis and therapy would be housed in the same device. Research into such technology is ongoing.[43,44]

Syncope

The role of remote monitoring in syncope is discussed elsewhere. However, potential future developments in physiologic sensors may allow for better methods of treating patients with recurrent syncope. For example, future sensors may allow for an alert system when a change in intravascular pressure or heart rate is sensed that may suggest an impending syncopal event. In addition, with advances in autonomic therapies, it may be possible to use therapeutic interventions to try to avert a syncopal event when changes in physiologic parameters suggest that one is impending.[45]

OTHER AREAS OF DEVELOPMENT

Other areas of development that are required are the continued miniaturization of technology and improved battery technology. It is possible that as more sensor options are available, the choice of sensors may need to be tailored to the patient. For example, a patient with heart failure may benefit from a different set of sensors and algorithms than a patient with recurrent syncope. In turn, novel uses of existing technology should be considered (such as using accelerometers already present in pacemakers and defibrillators to evaluate heart sounds) **(Fig. 4)**.[46]

To optimize use of a variety of sensors, batteries will also need to be improved to reduce the frequency of generator changes. Longer-lasting batteries may come at the expense of size, and both factors (battery life and device size) are critical aspects to the usefulness of future devices that use more complex technology.

POTENTIAL HURDLES

Large hurdles in the development of future monitoring technologies include battery life, data management, and cost. Battery life may be circumvented by improvements in battery technology. However, the quantity of data obtained will always be an issue and need to be reviewed by a live person. Even in the presence of an autofeedback system wherein the device is capable not only of sensing but also of effecting responses to physiologic changes, clinician input will always be needed.

The level at which the data need to be reviewed immediately versus accrued over time and evaluated at periodic office visits also needs to be considered. For example, in the case of invasive ambulatory blood pressure monitoring, changes in medications may be made based on a history of several weeks to a month of blood pressure trends. However, in the case of evolving volume overload in the setting of heart failure, more immediate intervention may be needed. At what level alerts implemented in the device can be used to advise the patient of the need to see a clinician needs to be clarified.

The cost of technological advancement also needs to be considered. The upfront cost of implantation of such technology may be high. Depending on the outcome sought, cost savings to the health care system may not be realized for

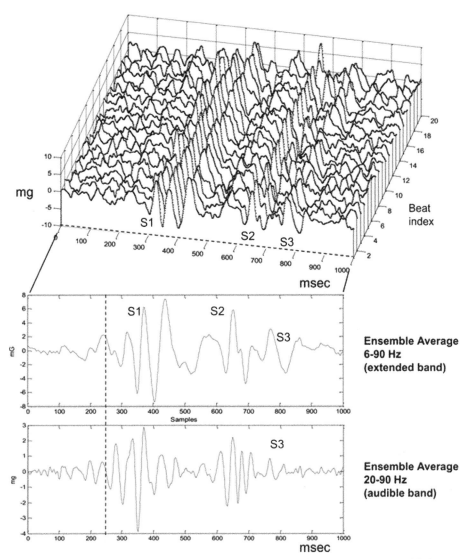

Fig. 4. How the accelerometer in a defibrillator may be used to assess for a third heart sound (S3) in patients with heart failure. R-wave aligned accelerometer traces are obtained from 20 consecutive beats (*top of figure*) and summed to create an ensemble average to attenuate noise. The frequency of the third heart sound in an inaudible extended band (*middle*) and in the audible band (*bottom*) can be seen relative to the other heart sounds using an algorithm to process the accelerometer data. (*From* Siejko KZ, Thakur PH, Maile K, et al. Feasibility of heart sounds measurements from an accelerometer within an ICD pulse generator. Pacing Clin Electrophysiol 2013;36(3):336; with permission.)

years or even decades. For example, in patients with heart failure, cost savings may be identified in terms of less frequent hospitalizations, and thus seen over the course of months to years. However, in the case of blood pressure monitoring, the cost value and clinical benefit of improved blood pressure control may not be seen for decades.

SUMMARY

Current monitoring technology is mostly aimed at either collecting and transmitting information about heart rate and rhythm or physiologic parameters that may suggest changes in heart failure status. The near future will likely see evolution in the use of wireless networks to transmit data more effectively as well as algorithms to improve the accuracy of arrhythmia recognition with available diagnostic monitors. Applications for smartphones have the potential to offer novel and cost-effective means by which to medically monitor patients as well. One key area of future development will be the evolution of physiologic sensors and effectors that can advance cardiac monitoring beyond heart rate and rhythm alone to other areas such as blood pressure monitoring, drug compliance and management, and treatments for syncope. However, the usefulness of any or all of these potential innovations will require extensive validation clinically as well as consideration of cost.

REFERENCES

1. Burri H, Heidbuchel H, Jung W, et al. Remote monitoring: a cost or an investment? Europace 2011; 13(Suppl 2):ii44–8.

2. Akematsu Y, Tsuji M. An empirical approach to estimating the effect of e-health on medical expenditure. J Telemed Telecare 2010;16:169–71.

3. Ricci RP, D'Onofrio A, Padeletti L, et al. Rationale and design of the health economics evaluation registry for remote follow up: TARIFF. Europace 2012; 14:1661–5.

4. Kapa S, Epstein AE, Callans DJ, et al. Assessing arrhythmia burden after catheter ablation of atrial fibrillation using an implantable loop recorder: the ABACUS Study. J Cardiovasc Electrophysiol 2013. http://dx.doi.org/10.1111/jce.12141. [Epub ahead of print].

5. Fernandez-Lopez H, Alfonso JA, Correia JH, et al. ZigBee-based remote patient monitoring. Stud Health Technol Inform 2012;177:229–34.

6. Grgic K, Zagar D, Krizanovic V. Medical applications of wireless sensor networks–current status and future directions. Med Glas (Zenica) 2012;9:23–31.

7. Rosenberg MA, Samuel M, Thosani A, et al. Use of a noninvasive continuous monitoring device in the management of atrial fibrillation: a pilot study. Pacing Clin Electrophysiol 2013;36:328–33.

8. Kinlay S, Leitch JW, Neil A, et al. Cardiac event recorders yield more diagnoses and are more cost-effective than 48-hour Holter monitoring in patients with palpitations. A controlled clinical trial. Ann Intern Med 1996;124:16–20.

9. Roche F, Gaspoz JM, Da Costa A, et al. Frequent and prolonged asymptomatic episodes of paroxysmal atrial fibrillation revealed by automatic long-term event recorders in patients with a negative 24-hour Holter. Pacing Clin Electrophysiol 2002;25: 1587–93.

10. Gula LJ, Krahn AD, Massel D, et al. External loop recorders: determinants of diagnostic yield in patients with syncope. Am Heart J 2004;147:644–8.

11. Lee YG, Jeong WS, Yoon G. Smartphone-based mobile health monitoring. Telemed J E Health 2012;18: 585–90.

12. Mosa AS, Yoo I, Sheets L. A systematic review of healthcare applications for smartphones. BMC Med Inform Decis Mak 2012;12:67.

13. McManus DD, Lee J, Maitas O, et al. A novel application for the detection of an irregular pulse using an iPhone 4S in patients with atrial fibrillation. Heart Rhythm 2013;10:315–9.

14. Pfaeffli L, Maddison R, Jiang Y, et al. Measuring physical activity in a cardiac rehabilitation population using a smartphone-based questionnaire. J Med Internet Res 2013;15(3):e61.

15. Nolan M, Mitchell JR, Doyle-Baker PK. Validity of the Apple iPhone/iPod Touch as an accelerometer-based physical activity monitor: a proof-of-concept study. J Phys Act Health 2013. [Epub ahead of print].

16. Kelly D, Caulfield B. An investigation into non-invasive physical activity recognition using smartphones. Conf Proc IEEE Eng Med Biol Soc 2012; 2012:3340–3.

17. Clifford GD, Clifton D. Wireless technology in disease management and medicine. Annu Rev Med 2012;63:479–92.

18. Basilakis J, Lovell NH, Redmond SJ, et al. Design of a decision-support architecture for management of remotely monitored patients. IEEE Trans Inf Technol Biomed 2010;14:1216–26.

19. Mokhtar MS, Basilakis J, Reedmond SJ, et al. A guideline-based decision support system for generating referral recommendations from routinely recorded home telehealth measurement data. Conf Proc IEEE Eng Med Biol Soc 2010; 2010:6166–9.

20. Boland P. The emerging role of cell phone technology in ambulatory care. J Ambul Care Manage 2007;30:126–33.

21. Lazarus A. Remote, wireless, ambulatory monitoring of implantable pacemakers, cardioverter defibrillators, and cardiac resynchronization therapy systems: analysis of a worldwide database. Pacing Clin Electrophysiol 2007;30:S2–12.

22. Parati G, Omboni S. Role of home blood pressure telemonitoring in hypertension management: an update. Blood Press Monit 2010;15:285–95.

23. Hindricks G, Pokushalov E, Urban L, et al. Performance of a new leadless implantable cardiac monitor in detecting and quantifying atrial fibrillation results of the XPECT trial. Circ Arrhythm Electrophysiol 2010;3:141–7.

24. Hong P, Sulke N. Implantable diagnostic monitors in the early assessment of syncope and collapse. Prog Cardiovasc Dis 2013;55:410–7.

25. McAdams E, Gehin C, Massot B, et al. The challenges facing wearable sensor systems. Stud Health Technol Inform 2012;177:196–202.

26. Eitel C, Husser D, Hindricks G, et al. Performance of an implantable automatic atrial fibrillation detection device: impact of software adjustments and relevance of manual episode analysis. Europace 2011; 13:480–5.

27. Arzbaecher R, Hampton DR, Burke MC, et al. Subcutaneous electrocardiogram monitors and their field of view. J Electrocardiol 2010;43:601–5.

28. Carter EV, Hickey KT, Pickham DM, et al. Feasibility and compliance with daily home electrocardiogram monitoring of the QT interval in heart transplant recipients. Heart Lung 2012;41:368–73.

29. Kaleschke G, Hoffmann B, Drewitz I, et al. Prospective, multicentre validation of a simple, patient-operated electrocardiographic system for the detection of arrhythmias and electrocardiographic changes. Europace 2009;11:1362–8.

30. Merchant FM, Dec GW, Singh JP. Implantable sensors for heart failure. Circ Arrhythm Electrophysiol 2010;3:657–67.

31. Zabel M, Vollmann D, Luthje L, et al. Randomized clinical evaluation of wireless fluid monitoring and remote ICD management using OptiVol alert-based predefined management to reduce cardiac decompensation and health care utilization: the CONNECT-OptiVol study. Contemp Clin Trials 2013;34:109–16.

32. Singh B, Russell SD, Cheng A. Update on device technologies for monitoring heart failure. Curr Treat Options Cardiovasc Med 2012;14:536–49.

33. Vanderheyden M, Houben R, Verstreken S, et al. Continuous monitoring of intrathoracic impedance and right ventricular pressures in patients with heart failure. Circ Heart Fail 2010;3:370–7.

34. O'Donoghue M, Braunwald E. Natriuretic peptides in heart failure: should therapy be guided by BNP levels? Nat Rev Cardiol 2010;7:13–20.

35. von Haehling S, Schefold JC, Lainscak M, et al. Inflammatory biomarkers in heart failure revisited: much more than innocent bystanders. Heart Fail Clin 2009;5:549–60.

36. Kanoupakis EM, Manios EG, Kallergis EM, et al. Serum markers of collagen turnover predict future shocks in implantable cardioverter-defibrillator recipients with dilated cardiomyopathy on optimal treatment. J Am Coll Cardiol 2010;55:2753–9.

37. Murphy OH, Bahmanyar MR, Borghi A, et al. Continuous in vivo blood pressure measurements using a fully implantable wireless SAW sensor. Biomed Microdevices 2013. http://dx.doi.org/10.1007/s10544-013-9759-7. [Epub ahead of print].

38. Tallaj JA, Singla I, Bourge RC. Implantable hemodynamic monitors. Heart Fail Clin 2009;5:261–70.

39. Potkay JA. Long term, implantable blood pressure monitoring systems. Biomed Microdevices 2008; 10:379–92.

40. Cong P, Young DJ, Hoit B, et al. Novel long-term implantable blood pressure monitoring system with reduced baseline drift. Conf Proc IEEE Eng Med Biol Soc 2006;1:1854–7.

41. Yang Q, Atanasov P, Wilkins E. A needle-type sensor for monitoring glucose in whole blood. Biomed Instrum Technol 1997;31:54–62.

42. Wang X, Mdingi C, DeHennis A, et al. Algorithm for an implantable fluorescence based glucose sensor. Conf Proc IEEE Eng Med Biol Soc 2012; 2012:3492–5.

43. Tao H, Kainerstorfer JM, Siebert SM, et al. Implantable, multifunctional, bioresorbable optics. Proc Natl Acad Sci U S A 2012;109:19584–9.

44. Nuxoll EE, Siegel RA. BioMEMS devices for drug delivery. IEEE Eng Med Biol Mag 2009;28:31–9.

45. Stavrakis S, Scherlag BJ, Po SS. Autonomic modulation: an emerging paradigm for the treatment of cardiovascular diseases. Circ Arrhythm Electrophysiol 2012;5:247–8.

46. Siejko KZ, Thakur PH, Maile K, et al. Feasibility of heart sounds measurements from an accelerometer within an ICD pulse generator. Pacing Clin Electrophysiol 2013;36(3):334–46.

Conclusions for *Cardiac Electrophysiology Clinics* Issue on Remote Monitoring and Physiologic Sensing Technologies

K.L. Venkatachalam, MD[a], Samuel J. Asirvatham, MD[b],*

KEYWORDS

- Remote monitoring • Cardiac implantable electronic device • Cardiac monitoring • Telemedicine
- Mobile cardiac outpatient telemetry

KEY POINTS

- Remote monitoring of cardiac parameters will continue to play an important clinical role in the diagnosis and treatment of cardiovascular disease.
- The volume of clinical data produced by the increasing use of this technology will need to be managed using efficient approaches to the processing of such data.
- The technologies will need to be thoroughly and continually tested in a clinical setting to confirm their relevance and to prevent clinicians being misled by the physiologic data.

As noted in this comprehensive issue, remote monitoring technologies are playing, and will continue to play, an increasingly important role in the management of patients with complex cardiac conditions. Indeed, the expansion of sensor technologies to include temperature, glucose, and other physiologic parameters may make these devices available and useful to a much wider patient population.

However, the enthusiasm regarding the availability of such technology must be tempered by the continued effort from relevant clinical studies and the concurrent development of sound evidence-based guidelines to support their use. This goal will also become harder to accomplish in practice, because the increased sophistication

and complexity of the algorithms needed to run such devices safely and effectively will probably result in longer review times for agency approvals (for clinical use), consequently longer development cycle times and, ultimately, a greater expense to the end user (the patient and the clinician).

Moreover, the potential for a dramatic increase in clinical data being generated by such devices cannot be underestimated. Even today, cardiac device clinic staff members face severe time constraints, with routine clinic checks, troubleshooting, and event-monitor analyses to be done on an expanding patient base. To prevent this from becoming an unmanageable burden, cardiac device companies must work in

Disclosures: The authors have nothing to disclose.

[a] Department of Internal Medicine, Division of Cardiovascular Diseases, Mayo Clinic Florida, 4500 San Pablo Road, Davis 7, Jacksonville, FL 32224, USA; [b] Department of Internal Medicine and Pediatric Cardiology, Saint Mary's Hospital, Mayo Clinic Minnesota, Mary Brigh Building 4-523, 1216 2nd Street Southwest, Rochester, MN 55902, USA

* Corresponding author.

E-mail address: asirvatham.samuel@mayo.edu

Card Electrophysiol Clin 5 (2013) 381–382
http://dx.doi.org/10.1016/j.ccep.2013.05.002

conjunction with clinicians on the front line, even during the early development phase of new technologies, to incorporate algorithms to streamline data gathering, electronic entry, and interpretation. Doing this as an afterthought would produce needless frustration for patients and clinicians, and may hamper the adoption of potentially useful technologies.

The user interface for patients and clinicians will also need to be simplified and made more intuitive to allow widespread use of these technologies by users with a broad range of experience with electronic devices. By streamlining all of the interfaces and easing the interpretation burden on the clinical staff, the overall cost to the consumer will also be minimized.

Index

Note: Page numbers of article titles are in **boldface** type.

A

Activity sensors
    for ICDs, 317–319
    for rate-adaptive pacing, 304–307
AF. *See* Atrial fibrillation (AF)
Atrial fibrillation (AF)
    asymptomatic
        remote monitoring for, 358–359
    described, 349–351
    incidence of, 349
    incidentally discovered by implanted pacemakers/
        defibrillators, 359–360
    prevalence of, 349, 357
    remote management of
        in patients with cardiac complaints
            ILRs for, 339
    remote monitoring for, 341, **357–364**
        evidence for, 358–361
            AF incidentally discovered by implanted
                pacemakers/defibrillators, 359–360
            asymptomatic AF, 358–359
            cryptogenic stroke, 360–361
            subclinical AF, 360–361
        Holter monitoring, 361
        introduction, 357
        management-related, 361–362
        options for, 357–358
        postablation, 362
        TTM, 361
1Atrial fibrillation (AF)
    in stroke and TIA patients
        significance of burden, 352–353
    subclinical
        remote monitoring for, 360–361

B

Biologic energy
    harvesting, 329–330
Biologic pacemaker, 331–334
Biomarker tracking and drug assays
    physiologic sensing in, 375–376
Blood pressure monitoring
    physiologic sensing in, 375

C

Cardiac monitoring
    remote
        history of, **275–282.** *See also* Remote cardiac
            monitoring
Cardiac pacing
    in patients with heart failure
        hemodynamic sensors for, 312–313
Cardiac rhythm monitoring
    devices for, 351–352
    remote
        state of the art in, 366–367
Chest pain
    remote monitoring of, 344
Closed-loop stimulation sensor
    for rate-adaptive pacing, 308–309
Cryptogenic stroke
    remote monitoring for, 360–361

D

Device and lead integrity monitoring
    state of the art in, 368
Drug delivery systems
    physiologic sensing in, 376
Dyspnea
    remote monitoring of, 341–343

E

Edema
    remote monitoring of, 341–343
Electrocardiogram (ECG)
    monitoring of
        beyond rate and rhythm
            in remote cardiac monitoring, 374

H

Heart failure
    cardiac pacing in patients with
        hemodynamic sensors for, 312–313
Heart failure monitoring
    physiologic sensing in, 375
    remote
        state of the art in, 367–368
Heart rate sensors
    for ICDs, 317–319
Hemodynamic sensors
    for cardiac pacing in patients with heart failure,
        312–313
Holter monitoring
    for AF, 361

Card Electrophysiol Clin 5 (2013) 383–385
http://dx.doi.org/10.1016/S1877-9182(13)00080-4
1877-9182/13/$ – see front matter © 2013 Elsevier Inc. All rights reserved.

Moving?

Make sure your subscription moves with you!

To notify us of your new address, find your **Clinics Account Number** (located on your mailing label above your name), and contact customer service at:

Email: journalscustomerservice-usa@elsevier.com

800-654-2452 (subscribers in the U.S. & Canada)
314-447-8871 (subscribers outside of the U.S. & Canada)

Fax number: 314-447-8029

Elsevier Health Sciences Division
Subscription Customer Service
3251 Riverport Lane
Maryland Heights, MO 63043

*To ensure uninterrupted delivery of your subscription, please notify us at least 4 weeks in advance of move.

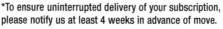

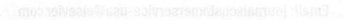

Printed and bound by CPI Group (UK) Ltd, Croydon, CR0 4YY

03/10/2024

01040301-0011